PRAISE FOR *BEYOND BEDRAILS AND BINGO*

"... a hands-on evaluation of an industry in desperate need of home improvement."

—BlueInk Review

"... a detailed and expansive survey of how nursing homes function in the United States."

—Foreword Reviews

"Libraries need to consider *Beyond Bedrails and Bingo* an essential addition as they stock quality books on healthcare, legal regulations, and consumer information."

—D. Donovan, Sr. Reviewer, *Midwest Book Review*

"*Beyond Bedrails and Bingo* reflected my experiences as a nurse who has spent four decades living through many of the situations Dave Devereaux describes...I wholeheartedly recommend {the book} as necessary reading for anyone who engages with the long-term care arm of the healthcare system."

—Robert A. Groves, *Readers' Favorite Reviews*

"Devereaux goes to great lengths to illustrate how, as a society, we are largely failing to care for our elderly, but he offers hope as well: great strides have been made in treatment and prevention, and medical advances are keeping loved ones out of nursing homes longer than previous generations."

—BookLife Review

"... a hard look at what we think we know about long-term care...Devereaux arms you with the tools to put you in a position of strength. Overall, this is an intelligent, detailed, and informative guide, and a must-have when making care home decisions. Very highly recommended."

—Jamie Michele, *Readers' Favorite*

"Dave Devereaux writes in a straightforward, conversational style that balances explanations with reflections, making complex industry topics easier to understand… It offers both information and perspective, encouraging readers to think about care, responsibility, and decision-making in meaningful ways."

—Carol Thompson, *Readers' Favorite Reviews*

BEYOND BEDRAILS *and* BINGO

Myths,
Truths, and
the Future
of America's
Nursing Homes

DAVE DEVEREAUX

Beyond Bedrails and Bingo: Myths, Truths, and the Future of America's Nursing Homes
Published by Layton Road Press
Eatonton, GA

Names: Devereaux, Dave, author.
Title: Beyond bedrails and bingo : myths, truths, and the future of America's nursing homes / Dave Devereaux.
Description: Eatonton, GA : Layton Road Press, [2026] | Includes bibliographical references.
Identifiers: ISBN: 9798994220009 (paperback) | 9798994220016 (hardcover) | 9798994220023 (ebook)
Subjects: LCSH: Nursing homes--United States. | Long-term care facilities--United States. | Older people--Care--United States. | Medical care--United States. | Older people--Care--United States--Decision making. | Population aging--United States. | Nursing homes--United States--Management. | Medical policy--United States. | Health care reform--United States. | Kinship care--United States. | Caregivers--United States. | BISAC: HEALTH & FITNESS / Health Care Issues. | BUSINESS & ECONOMICS / Industries / Healthcare.
Classification: LCC: RA997 .D48 2026 | DDC: 362.16/0973--dc23

Cover design by Laura Duffy Design, copyright owned by Dave Devereaux.
Cover photograph: iStock/love portrait and love the world
Interior formatting by Asya Blue Design, copyright owned by Dave Devereaux.
Author photograph: Andrew Thayer, Temple University

Disclaimer:
This book is intended for informational and educational purposes only. It does not constitute legal, medical, financial, or professional advice. The experiences, insights, and opinions expressed are those of the author and are based on personal experience within the long-term care industry. While care has been taken to ensure accuracy, the practices, regulations, and policies governing nursing homes and elder care vary by state and are subject to change. Readers should consult qualified professionals regarding specific situations or decisions related to elder care, healthcare, or long-term care planning.

QUANTITY PURCHASES: Schools, companies, professional groups, clubs, and other organizations may qualify for special terms when ordering quantities of this title.
For information, go to: davedevereaux.com

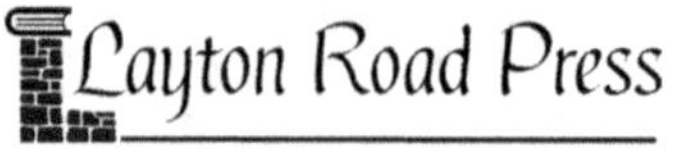

CONTENTS

FOREWORD

America's nursing homes are facing challenges that could determine their very survival—and few understand those challenges better than my mentor, Dave Devereaux.

Thirty-eight years ago, I was a young administrator at a small skilled nursing facility in Wisconsin. I gave a presentation entitled "The Crisis in Care." My message was simple: While the issues were many, three stood out as especially urgent: overregulation, limited staffing, and poor reimbursement.

Today, as a nursing home owner and operator of North Shore Health, I can't help but ask myself: *Have we made any difference?* because it seems we are facing those very same challenges today. For too long, our profession has played defense instead of offense. We respond to negative press, complain about low Medicaid rates, and argue that regulations are excessive and often miss the mark. In doing so, we allow others to dictate our fate.

With years of experience in the field and Dave's guidance, one thing has been made abundantly clear: Nobody can tell our story, advocate for our staff and residents, or shape our future better than those who live it every day. If the industry wants to survive and thrive, we must start telling that story ourselves.

I am honored to introduce you to this debut book by my esteemed mentor, Dave Devereaux, *Beyond Bedrails and Bingo: Myths, Truths, and the Future of America's Nursing Homes*. Throughout his decorated career, Dave has consistently delivered exceptional results and built a stellar reputation in our profession. His common-sense, real-world approach to business resonates with everyone he leads, making him a trusted advisor to many.

By creating a culture that attracts and retains great leaders, educates consumers, and builds long-term relationships with legislators and regulators, providers can achieve lasting success. Never has this been more critical than it is today, which is why I believe *Beyond Bedrails and Bingo* is a must-read.

True to Dave's leadership approach, this book does not gloss over the hard realities of our profession. Some days are incredibly rewarding while others bring challenges that feel almost insurmountable. He makes it clear that there are no shortcuts to success—no "easy button." Our field is continually evolving. Those who succeed adopt a "no excuses" mindset, take calculated risks, and position their organizations for both today and the future.

Beyond Bedrails and Bingo, which he dedicated to improving the lives of seniors, is filled with experiences, best practices, and lessons learned throughout Dave's career. He even incorporates a couple of his passions to help tell this important story. For music and sports enthusiasts—enjoy.

I recently asked Dave why he chose to write such a comprehensive account of his experiences. He replied quickly and without hesitation: "It would be a real shame if I didn't use this knowledge to give back and help others. If done right, it will help our profession and improve patient care." That is a true leader and mentor.

Unfortunately, many nursing homes have already closed their doors, and promising leaders have left our profession. The reality is that more closures and departures are likely in the coming years. But Dave provides a detailed roadmap showing why it doesn't have to be that way.

I am confident *Beyond Bedrails and Bingo* will educate, challenge, and inspire readers just as Dave has inspired so many throughout his career. As you move through these pages, I hope you'll find the clarity and confidence needed to navigate the challenges ahead and shape a stronger future for our field.

David M. Mills
Managing Director, North Shore Health
Milwaukee, Wisconsin
November 2025

PREFACE

I remember my first trip to a nursing home. It was in 1966.

My mom, a registered nurse, was the home's evening supervisor, and my brothers and I had to spend a few hours there until her shift ended. It was after supper, and people living there walked the halls, received evening medications, and got ready for bed.

In an empty room, directly across from the nursing station, we didn't dare make a sound. With the door cracked, we saw everything happening at the station until the hallway lights dimmed, and most people went to their own rooms.

Quite an experience for a four-year-old.

Twelve years later, after countless visits back to that same building, I took a summer job as a housekeeper. It was a life-changing experience.

The building, originally the Pennsylvania Coal Co. headquarters, displayed *the largest piece of anthracite ever brought to the Earth's surface* at its entrance. Mammoth in size and substance, its interior was retrofitted to take advantage of the new Medicare and Medicaid programs enacted in the mid-sixties.

Three floors of rooms, ranging in size from single-bed to four-person wards, served 180 patients. Community bathrooms were standard on each floor—one per gender, with three stalls and two sinks each. There was a common dining and activity area on each floor.

There was no air conditioning.

I *loved* being there.

After summers of hanging out and watching television with my brothers, cutting grass, swimming at a local pool, bullshitting with my best friend, or waiting until it was time to go to baseball practice or a game, this wasn't eight fifty-minute classroom periods in which to learn, spread over 180 days, only to be interrupted by another ninety days of game shows, reruns, and ballgames. This learning differed from everything I'd ever known.

I got paid too.

Not much, but more than previous summers—$2.35 an hour. I learned about state and federal taxes. To me, as a sixteen-year-old kid, that seemed a total rip-off.

For the next three summers, and every weekend and holiday in-between, I worked in that nursing home. I came to know and enjoy the company of many patients and created lasting friendships with coworkers.

Other pursuits, *except for baseball*—my first love—fell to the wayside, and were replaced with the opportunity to learn, earn, and be something different. While hardworking classmates chucked newspapers in front yards, grilled and fried fast food, pumped gas, shagged hay for a local farmer, or volunteered, I experienced sights, sounds, and smells in a classroom that high school could never replicate.

My experiences were *stories*, involving different people who were interesting, funny, sad, and memorable.

As examples, I tried my high school Spanish out on Carmen, a patient whose grandson was a local middleweight and a damn good fighter. Her Spanish was better than mine. Much.

Rosie was in constant motion, talking about Orlando, or Yolanda, not knowing if they were the same person, or family members deep in her memory. When clean clothes came out of the laundry, she'd help sort and fold.

John was a longtime patient, beloved by all, as was Jimmy, uncle to two of my high school classmates and brother to my high school librarian. John had a girlfriend in town and spent many evenings (and early mornings) in undisclosed locations and beer gardens.

To these people, and many others, I owed thanks for helping me understand the absolute—as opposed to relative—value of living, the adventure of aging, and the brevity of life itself.

What incredible lessons to learn as a teenager.

ఌ

My mother, promoted years earlier to director of nursing, carried great responsibility and demanded respect. Watching her work in a leadership role was just like the experience of being at home. Mom was the boss, and was in control until she was out of control. As a kid, taking care of business in school or on the field meant life was good. As an employee, the bar remained high, with similar consequences. Exacting standards were routinely applied. When met, and even when not, best and honest effort was appreciated. For her, being in charge and making decisions was routine and familiar. I took direction and counsel from her, at work and at home, and am grateful for these lifelong gifts.

Throughout college and graduate school, I had many jobs I didn't love, and they didn't love me back. Every time I spent any time thinking or talking about what I wanted to be when I grew up, the only two answers I could honestly accept were: baseball coach and nursing home administrator.

Since coaching would only be a part-time solution to paying lifelong, everyday bills, becoming an administrator became my chosen career path. Spending my life doing anything else didn't seem to fit. I was very young and loved being around old people and those that cared for them.

My friends thought I was nuts. Not many people get up each morning and say … "I can't wait to work in a nursing home!"

After passing the state and federal examinations required to become a licensed nursing home administrator, I was hired as an assistant administrator of a home, located just outside of Philadelphia. Three months later, the home's administrator resigned without notice, and I was put in charge. From that day on, the world moved quickly, and has never seemed to stop.

Over the next forty years, I would …

… live in seventeen different homes, in nine states.

… work as a nursing home administrator in three homes in two different states.

… work for three publicly held, for-profit healthcare companies, each of which was sold, merged, or was the target of a hostile takeover.

… be promoted from supervising a single nursing home to overseeing an organization with over 700 nursing homes and assisted living facilities in thirty-eight states.

… have responsibility for overseeing the opening of newly constructed facilities; the closure of facilities with performance problems, an aging physical plant, or a shrinking market; the expansion of facilities with greater opportunity; and the integration of facilities via merger or acquisition.

… observe the love and commitment of countless families toward someone for whom they cared deeply.

… endure the actions of people who left a family member on a nursing home's doorstep and later argued about "needing" that family member's Social Security check.

… experience the celebration that accompanies a home earning statewide or national recognition for excellence in patient care.

… suffer the embarrassment and frustration that accompanied family members filing patient care lawsuits.

… watch people grow and advance in their careers, improving their own lives and their families.

... participate in the development of very talented people whose career paths eventually culminated in C-suite (chief executive or chief operating officer) roles within nursing home companies.

... experience the full spectrum of human emotion and behavior during four lasting moments in contemporary history—the AIDS epidemic, 9/11, Hurricane Katrina, and the COVID pandemic.

... watch people leave the industry, vowing never to return, and others, full of enthusiasm and desire, possessing big hearts and skilled hands entering to take their own turn.

... and experience the unimaginable challenge of admitting my mom to a nursing home.

ᘓ

Over the years, I've also been able to do some other—and different—things.

I've given back—endowing a chair in the Department of Nursing where I attended graduate school, recognizing and celebrating Mom's fifty years as a nurse. A source of great pride, this was a public way to thank someone that I loved and trusted.

I've put my time, energy, and money into a project designed to improve the assessment and treatment of pressure injuries, commonly referred to as bed sores. Among nursing homes using this project, incredible results are occurring.

I've spent time in the courtroom, providing expert testimony in patient-care-related cases, for both plaintiffs and defendants.

With a very good friend and college classmate as a partner, I launched and operated a business transporting people to medical appointments, many of whom were patients in a nursing home or assisted living facility.

What I have not yet done is share the experiences of my profession in a way that will benefit others.

While referring to this as a profession, it's also a lifestyle. A lifestyle I chose and embraced, spanning parts of six decades. In spending the last few years preparing, researching, and writing this book, this profession and lifestyle continues.

Given the choice, I wouldn't trade it for another.

At the same time, this profession, industry, and lifestyle is not easily understood by many.

Until now.

ꕤ

In these next ten chapters, I will share information not easily acquired from outside the nursing home business. Candidly, upon finishing this book, you'll possess a wider knowledge base and deeper understanding of complex, important topics than many who've spent years in this profession.

Providers of care will go by many names, including nursing homes, long-term-care centers, rehabilitation facilities and other labels constructed over decades of discussions among branding experts, marketing executives, and policymakers. In the context of this book, I'll generally use the phrase "nursing home," as in many cases it is *the home* where people live and receive care, with *nursing* as the primary service being delivered.

Partly due to fear of the unknown, nursing homes are often viewed as *America's Nightmare*. We'll examine the nature and causes of these fears and demystify common—and sometimes, strongly-held—impressions about this framework of healthcare, which recently celebrated its sixtieth anniversary as a *big* business.

We'll explore the people and their behaviors—in private and public sector roles—in this rapidly approaching $1 trillion industry.

And we'll follow the money, and it's linkages to incentivized behaviors.

Finally, we'll evaluate emerging trends and influencers, and options which exist today—on a small scale—and others anticipated to change the way we behave around getting older and remaining independent.

Portions of this book will surprise. Others will challenge tradition and convention. A few may conflict with values. Building knowledge relies on provoking thought, stimulating a desire to look beyond the information shared, and pursuing a deeper understanding.

We'll do this intentionally. The subject of taking care of people unable to take care of themselves—writ large—is complex and incredibly emotional. Historically, it's been poorly communicated and, as a result, frequently misunderstood.

Until now.

ᔓ

I will make you this promise: when you've finished this book, you will:

- Know more about the players in the nursing home world and how the myriad of pieces fit together
- Think differently about yourself, your future care needs, and the needs of those around you
- Act differently when discussing the topics of aging, care options, and roles and responsibilities as adult child, mother, father, sister, or brother
- Talk differently to people who matter in your life about tomorrow, and the days, months, years, and decades ahead
- Feel differently about your ability to influence—and control—where you live, what you do, and who takes care of you
- Behave differently as a result of knowing things that you might not have known before
- Possess confidence in the questions you'll ask, and things to look and listen for, when evaluating what's best for you and those you love

I hope you enjoy every word.

I

MANY PEOPLE ARE AFRAID OF NURSING HOMES

"Promise me you'll never put me in a nursing home. Promise."

If you've ever had someone look you squarely in the eyes and say this—as I have—your heart immediately breaks. Twice.

Promise.

The first occurs as they ask for your promise. If you've been seated beside someone trying to squeeze their final few hours, minutes, or seconds out of living, you'll know this look of fear.

Promise.

The second, and concurring, heartbreak is realizing that among the variables we truly believe are within our control, there are equally as many that make keeping this promise impossible.

Promise.

And as this impossible promise is made, fear grabs you and squeezes the breath from your body.

Promise.

ᔕ

Why do people ask for this promise?

Would you ever want to live in a nursing home? Not until you felt you had no other choice, I'll bet.

Many times, people will do anything possible to avoid one. Why? Take a minute and think of your own reasons.

For me, I like my independence and would prefer to keep it. Still, there is a second reason for people not wanting to live in a nursing home. *Living in a nursing home is hard.* It's very hard.

At the time of this writing, the Kaiser Family Foundation estimates that approximately 1.2 million Americans live in a nursing home.[1] People likely didn't choose this willingly. Circumstances which directly threatened their safety or existence drove these choices.

Places where I'm most comfortable, excluding my own home, include:

- Baseball fields where tickets don't require a smartphone
- Classrooms and lecture halls where people pay attention
- Bars where bartenders wash glasses, talk to customers, and double as bouncer
- Nursing homes

Yep, nursing homes. After being in, around, and through over a *thousand* nursing homes, and working over a *hundred thousand* hours on behalf of these homes, it's like being at the ballpark, in class, or elbows down on hardwood.

But I wouldn't like to live in one. It wouldn't be home.

People—as Patients

Conversations about nursing homes should center around the people being cared for. Without them, nursing homes don't remain nursing homes.

During the 1990s, my employer conducted a study to determine how people living in a nursing home defined themselves. This became important work, as inconsistencies in how company employees referred to those being cared for were creating hard feelings and inconsistency in departmental and company-wide communication.

This study uncovered that people being cared for in our nursing homes defined themselves as patients. Not customers, guests, clients, or residents.

Patients.

Respondents shared that because they were under a doctor's care, seen daily by nurses and nursing assistants for their needs, and were unable to care for themselves, they were patients.

And, unsurprisingly, no one considered "this place" as their home.

For this book, I'll refer to people being cared for in a nursing home as patients. During my career, I chose to respect patients' wishes whenever possible.

Yes, on its surface, this may appear trivial. We know, however, that words do matter.

A Shared Sentiment

A ba-zillion dollar research grant from the National Institutes of Health (NIH) isn't needed to figure this out. When asked, nursing home patients will tell you the same.

Fear. A four-letter word as powerful as it is austere.

A patient's fear of a nursing home is completely understandable. When entering a nursing home, it's nothing close to the experience of checking into a hotel or visiting family or friends. Without fail, something traumatic has happened to this person, requiring hospitalization and treatment, before transferring to the nursing home.

Something awful, scary, and life-changing.

This trauma may be linked to an event. A fall. Major surgery. A chronic condition that can't be managed safely elsewhere. Losing the help of others, which enabled them to live at home.

No matter what, this surprise occurred very quickly, resulting in changes they weren't prepared for.

Imagine if something like this happened to you. Would you feel nervous or anxious? How about scared? Or even, terrified?

Now, let's further explore this person's trauma.

Consider their experience of falling at home and breaking a hip. With sensitivity to the associated pain and anxiety, this is a minimum of what the person might endure:

- A period of overwhelming pain and helplessness
- A 911 call
- A seemingly interminable wait for help
- The embarrassment of EMS (and police) arriving at your home
- Being placed on a gurney—by strangers
- Being placed in an ambulance—by the same strangers
- Being driven to a hospital
- Transferring from one gurney to another
- Waiting, secured to the gurney, staring at the ceiling, unfamiliar voices everywhere
- Fielding more questions than imaginable, quickly—by new strangers
- Treatment, including the possibility of surgery—by even newer strangers
- Laying in fear for hours wondering, *What's going to happen to me?*

The experiential summary for the person falling and breaking a hip would encompass several pages more and *is* an example of what they endure *before* entering a nursing home. Once becoming a patient, their experiential summary lengthens, including:

- *More* strangers
- *More* questions
- *More* worries

From the time of the fall—and each day in a nursing home—this patient's life will be full of:

- **Unfamiliar people.** Nurses, nursing assistants, therapists, physicians, department heads, and people in charge. Without a scorecard, it's almost impossible to keep up with the names, faces, roles, and stories behind these people.

  And for *these people*, it will be almost impossible to keep up with stories about this patient.

  While there can be hundreds of people who work in, live in, and visit a nursing home each day, for a patient, it can be the loneliest place on Earth. Familiar faces and routine activities from their lives are replaced with confusion, a loss of control, and a lack of independence.

- **Questions.** About bills to be paid, family and friends, the roommate in the next bed, the customary glass of wine with dinner, or the dog left at home. Questions about care and everything else, while important, are secondary.

  For these questions, it's almost impossible to provide complete or satisfactory answers. For this patient, their fear of the unknown will be real and constant.

- **Worries.** About completely recovering from their injury, being forgotten by others, and not being able to have prized possessions within view or reach.

  Further compounding these worries is the patient confronting their own mortality. Not only due to this fall, but ones that most likely will occur in their future. Their frequent, inescapable worry—*Is this the beginning of the end for me?*

Last, from the time of the fall—and each day living in a nursing home—the life of this patient will be consumed with a question and worry that dominates their attention.

When can I go home?

It's natural, and expected that nearly every nursing home patient wants to go home. If we were in similar situations, we would want this.

Each day, nursing home patients across the nation return home. People improve, reaching the point where returning home is very much the right thing. This is cause for celebration, recognizing that good things can—and do—happen in nursing homes. This fact may be lost, or simply unknown. Nevertheless, it happens.

Until this occurs, patients are consumed with their realities. Pain and fear. Loneliness and isolation.

Losing Too Much

Take ten seconds to think about the daily or weekly pleasures you're in control of. Things you enjoy. A cigarette with your morning coffee? A Diet Coke or Mountain Dew? Dinner delivered? Or is a Starbucks something needed to fully function?

When your day's done, do you pour two fingers of Old No. 7, grab a Bud or a glass of wine, or stop at a place to hang with friends and neighbors?

If you have the time, resources, and independence to enjoy indulgences like these, you're lucky. We each have our own lists of life's simple pleasures, and they help us celebrate the start (or finish) of another day or week. Without them, life's meaning would become emptier.

Small things make a big difference.

Now, imagine that all these simple pleasures were taken away because you:

- Lost your health
- Lost your mobility or independence

- Lost your home
- Lost your income or wealth

Some of these losses could be gradual. You don't get around as well as before, or you lost confidence in driving. Rent went up. The Social Security check doesn't cover the inflated prices of food and other essentials you've depended on.

Your memory, changing gradually, now threatens your safety. Family and friends that you leaned on for support are gone, or are no longer able to give due to their own personal challenges.

As control of these pleasures fades or is taken away, your approach to everyday living depends on the calendar, timetable, and rules made by others—strangers.

Losing both control and life's simple pleasures would suck. For nursing home patients, it absolutely does too, further compounding their fears.

One Very Long Night

As a nursing home administrator, sensitivity training about the patient experience seemed endless. As more becomes known about aging and disability, more is shared. The impact of one training was especially long-lasting.

For ninety minutes, we had to perform numerous sensory and environmental alterations, including:

- Removing jackets, sweaters, shoes, and eyeglasses
- Getting comfortable with the room temperature being set to 60º F
- Filling a pair of bedroom slippers with marbles and putting them on
- Inserting cotton balls in each ear

- Smearing petroleum jelly across the lenses of a pair of eyeglasses and wearing them
- Wearing a pair of cloth gloves, whose fingers had popsicle sticks or tongue depressors affixed at varying lengths
- Resuming attention to the training's instructor, who gave zero consideration to these alterations

The temperature drop creates a change in metabolism and blood circulation. It sucks being cold.

The marble-laden slippers simulated the sensation of foot ailments. It hurts like hell to walk on marbles.

The cotton balls simulated auditory deficits. It's tough to hear anything with your ears stuffed.

The eyeglasses simulated altered visual acuity. Rain-X wouldn't clear this blurred visual field.

The gloves simulated altered joint function and fine motor skills deficits. Eating, writing, and grasping are miserable when your hands and fingers don't work.

If you've experienced this type of training—or have these conditions—you can relate.

Academy Award-winning actress Bette Davis, who lived to age eighty-one, may have put it best:[2] "Getting old isn't for sissies." Truer words were never spoken. This training made me a believer. It's tough getting old.

Several years later, I was overseeing more than a hundred nursing homes and assisted living facilities across several states and time zones. With no two locations being alike, the goal was to provide the best possible patient care experience in each.

With this in mind, I wanted to experience twenty-four hours in a nursing home and apply this learning to my work. Fully appreciating that this wouldn't equate to the patient's reality of living in a home, it was closer than I'd ever been before.

The first time I'd ever visited this nursing home was earlier the same day. With the administrator's approval and knowledge limited to a few members of the nursing home management team, I entered the building via wheelchair late one evening, occupying an empty semiprivate room. I was going to be a short-term patient, almost exclusively bedbound, and recovering from a hospital stay. I brought:

- No identification
- No clothes or personal items
- No money, phone, or electronic devices
- No reading material or food

I told no one where I was.

I was given a hospital gown, and I got into bed. It was late and most every other patient was in bed.

My most vivid memories from this experience were:

- At night, it never got dark.
- Day or night, it was never quiet.
- People entered my room frequently.
- Almost no one asked me my name.
- Those who did didn't ask much more.

Several patients walked or wheeled themselves into my room during the day. Some came right up to the head of the bed. A few asked questions, and a few more made themselves comfortable.

The food was OK. I really wanted a beer.

I was completely alone with my thoughts. This was a new experience.

At the end of the twenty-four hours, someone came into my room, gave me the clothes I'd worn the previous day, and wheeled me out of the patient care area. I grabbed the keys to my rental car and returned to the hotel I'd been staying at during this trip.

On the way to the hotel, I stopped and grabbed a quart of Budweiser. Entering my room, I opened my quart of Bud and turned on ESPN. I didn't hear a single word said while watching SportsCenter. One thought lived inside my head. *Living in a nursing home is hard. If I ever really had to, I'd be afraid too.*

Families Don't Get a Pass

A family's fears about nursing homes, while understandable, are more complex than that of their loved one. As my mother's power of attorney for healthcare and finances during her care in a home, complex feelings remain, more than a year after her death.

For starters, family members sometimes suffer from misplaced embarrassment when choosing to place their loved one in a home. Unshakable self-doubt and the slings and arrows of friends and neighbors can be endless. Explaining or defending the reasons for this choice is equally difficult.

Their frequent and silent thought (mine too) ... *I'm afraid I made a mistake.*

Long-standing beliefs that *nothing would ever change* results in accumulated unchecked family baggage. Things done and undone. Said and unsaid. Time spent on things that didn't matter, or never would, with people that you thought mattered and never really did.

Distance—proximal and personal—which resulted in missing the things that ended up mattering a whole lot more than you originally thought. Saying *no* to things you should have been saying *yes* to all along. These unresolved issues, unshared secrets, and unspoken sentiments make everything harder.

They also make family members afraid. Afraid that time is running out. Afraid that life's accumulated baggage will remain unchecked.

During a loved one's nursing home stay, family members sometimes resent the time spent searching, organizing, understanding, and executing unattended business on behalf of their loved one. Understandably, it's time taken away from *other* things—work, play, rest, friends. The very things they might have been told they weren't to do when younger.

When siblings are involved—especially those living out-of-town—local family members frequently own every perceived (and real) shortcoming associated with their loved one's care. Distant sisters and brothers judge health states, care provided, and the home selected. For family members most present with a patient, it's a heavy responsibility. Carrying this weight can result in a domestic throwdown.

In a number of cases, however, the prospect of family members becoming separated from their loved one's money results in anxiety—or anger. Families relying on monthly income from their loved one's Social Security or pension may find this money no longer available once the patient enters a home.

These unpleasantries are because this money—Social Security or monthly pension—had been used to pay the rent or mortgage, utilities, or food—for themselves and their family. In their world, they *needed* this money. On occasion, frightened family members have gasped, "Well then, what am I going to live on?"

In other cases, families unfamiliar with the price of nursing home care experience massive sticker shock. Out-of-pocket costs can be hundreds daily and several thousand monthly. Money paid to a nursing home can quickly whittle away at the amounts available for inheritance. Family members can (and will) count, treating amounts paid for care as future financial losses to them.

Predictably, these dynamics can consume family members. And among family members where *none* of these reasons apply, this last one is primal, powerful, and unavoidable: Family members become scared.

Contrary to others, this point doesn't use the word "may." Fear enters everyone's emotional equation. Scared—of pain and suffering, feeling alone, or having to live their own first and future days without a person that they've probably known since birth.

One's mortality is no longer an abstraction. It's an open-handed slap in the face.

Embracing this reality is hard. It just is.

This realization—my mom's admission and stay in a nursing home, followed by memory care—frightened me. Recognizing that the future could never be the same as the past, memories would likely fade, and the present would become a painful, lasting memory was scary.

For a while, I was afraid:

- For Mom. I knew what was ahead for her and what she'd lost. I feared for how the seesaw of intermittent reminiscences would affect her, and how I'd handle experiencing these highs and lows.
- For my daughters, who'd feel Mom's absence at graduations, weddings, and the arrival of their own children.
- For my nieces and nephews, who'd have similar life experiences with rich stories and memories.
- For myself, as she was my biggest fan and harshest critic, and the truest source of unconditional love, and wouldn't be a part of anything—for the first time in nearly sixty years.

Though these fears have abated, they'll never be erased. This is the experience of being a patient's family member.

Anger Management

As a patient's stay lengthens, a family member's contempt for the nursing home often follows.

Role reversal, in which the parent (now, patient) is viewed as childlike by their adult child, who is now serving as parent and decision-maker—by force or choice—contributes to this distress.

These transitions aren't always smooth. The patient, trying desperately to maintain their independence and self-determination, will resist infantilization by their adult children, resulting in hard feelings or willful behavior when out of sight. Who can blame them? Are any of us really ready for the days our kids make the rules?

With limited options and waning prospects for returning home, patients, when able, will push boundaries in familiar areas, including alcohol, tobacco, food preferences, new relationships, and sex. Yes. Like we probably did as teenagers. Patients want life beyond the dining room and rehab gym.

The adult child—wrestling with embarrassment, regret, anger, fear—is reluctant to unload on their loved one. Eye rolling, hyperventilating, and head shaking will do. Risking being thought of as unkind or abusive to an old, sick, or injured person is intolerable.

Yet value or virtue collisions involving drinking, smoking, swearing, eating things that aren't good for them, associating with "unsavory" people, or consorting with members of the same or opposite sex "must be addressed."

These demands result from the adult child becoming parent ... to their parent. The things I heard most from adult children were:

- They're too old.
- They don't know what they're doing.
- That should have ended when Mom (or Dad) died.
- Mom's (or Dad's) behavior is making me uncomfortable.
- They (the adult child) shouldn't have to talk to Mom (or Dad) about what is making them uncomfortable.

This results in family members searching for places to deposit their anger. Anger, sown from their own fears and anxieties.

Because their loved one's care and safety is dependent on the efforts of nurses and nursing assistants, families won't channel their innermost

Shirley MacLaine (think, *Terms of Endearment*) toward the people at the nursing station. It is too risky.

Instead, they will transfer their fears and anxieties—with speed and accuracy—toward the home's administrator.

Why? For starters, there aren't other targets for family members to rip.

And family members know that administrators *must* take it. They know that administrators won't fire back. Reputations, jobs, and careers are at risk if they do.

Yet, an administrator's ability to influence changes requested by family members only goes so far. Especially when it involves residents' rights, which indicates that nursing home patients are provided choice, respect, and dignity—across a host of topics—and those rights can't be violated by the nursing home or a patient's family member.

When family members are confronted with the word NO—for anything, in the name of residents' rights—anger is instantly directed toward the nursing home's administrator.

Yes. Anger. Family members don't like being told "No." Families of nursing home patients can dish out anger like they're pursuing an Olympic gold medal.

They'll mock administrators, mimicking their voice pattern or word choice, repeating everything said, in the precise manner stated.

Using an industry term—or one not readily understood—in a conversation invites family member retorts with extra emphasis, inviting you to choke on whatever word you've uttered.

Families will sometimes anoint an administrator with a nickname, based on physical features which engender amusement or derision.

- Shorter administrators might be known as Sawed-Off or Shorty.
- Taller administrators might be known as Stretch or Olive Oyl.

- Wearing a cross or other religious adornment also qualifies as fair game.

Everything is fair game. Pictures in the office. The car driven to work. The shade of lipstick. Creative families can string together a nickname like a mathematical equation.

Mustache + East Coast Heritage = That Frito Bandito, Yankee Bastard

OK, now you know *my* administrator nickname among family members at one of my ports of call.

Yeah. Anger. Sown from their own completely understandable fears and anxieties.

Conflicting Expectations and Inevitabilities

Excepting for instances when patients recover and return home, nursing homes and patients' attending physicians are expected to consistently meet these constant, invisible standards implied by family members:

- Regardless of a patient's age, illness, or infirmity, they're *never* supposed to die.
- Nothing bad should *ever* happen.

For families, watching change occur in someone they love—freedom, function, interests, and enjoyment lost, increased pain, fear, loneliness, regret—is excruciating. It's visible. Heartbreakingly so. It's real, and really awful. And families don't want to acknowledge it.

So they don't. They cling to this invisible and implied standard, using it as a club to beat back fears and anxieties associated with their own guilt, anger, or regret. Nursing home leadership, nurses, caregivers, and physicians aren't spared.

These thoughts aren't a product of observing others. My experiences involving family members—across four generations—helped me move from believing people were *never* supposed to die … to not supposed to die *this soon* … or supposed to die *this way*—to believing that it does indeed happen to all of us—and that itself is *never* a surprise.

Talking about dying is hard. Talking to patients about dying is harder.

It's something that few ever become any good at. Everyday people, nursing home leaders, and doctors grapple with this dynamic.

Yes, doctors. In moments of candor, doctors will share that they're really bad in talking about someone dying. A bestselling and award-winning book, *Being Mortal: Medicine and What Matters in the End,* by Atul Gawande[3], tells a compelling story about this topic.

Inevitably, a person's illness and underlying condition falls short of the invisible, implied standard of family members, elevating fears and anxieties, resulting in many of the dynamics shared throughout this chapter.

This inevitability sometimes involves a phenomenon witnessed in nursing home patients. Expressed as a sentence, it is: Sick people get sick of being sick.

When reaching this point, patients seem to respond to an internal voice saying, *"I quit!"* and the beginning of their end begins.

Visible signs include:

- Meals previously consumed fully go half eaten.
- Medications previously taken on time and without dispute are rejected or spit out.
- Therapy appointments that were religiously attended are refused.
- Repositioning to prevent skin breakdown … is undone once caregivers leave the room.

Many times, these acts are made by patients who are no longer afraid of a nursing home. No more strangers, questions, or worries. After having lost almost everything, they've resumed control over the remainder of time on their life's clock.

ᔓᔕ

As readers, your introduction to reasons why people are afraid of nursing homes is complete. While knowledge and understanding won't permanently extinguish them, you are well prepared to examine more complex and provocative topics involving people—patients, family members, nursing home workers and caregivers, and others—with a vested, or central, interest in matters involving nursing homes.

For most of the remaining chapters, a section serves as a summary of topics you can ask about, or look and listen for, applying your growing knowledge base and deeper understanding about how things work and the roles played by people involved.

WHAT YOU CAN DO

Ask Questions About:

- Unchecked baggage with loved ones. What can (or should) be done to "'check" it?
- Ownership for decision-making with out-of-town siblings. Will armchair quarterbacking from others influence your choices? Or cause you to second-guess?
- Financial matters. Is a family member dependent on a loved one's savings, pension, or Social Security?
- What your loved ones are most afraid of. Who can help overcome these fears?
- Your own fears. What's causing them, and what can you do about them?

Look for:

- Options. For everything that matters. Problems have more than one solution. Is there enough time, money, and help to create an expansive menu of options?
- Help. Pride and ego aren't your friends. Small favors can yield big returns.

Listen to What People Say:

- Is your loved one giving you signs that they are sick of being sick?

II

THE DISRESPECT FOR NURSING HOME PATIENTS IS AN OPEN SECRET

"Never mind what people tell you. Watch what they do."

When I was a kid, parents, coaches, and teachers gave me this advice. Simple. Practical. Deep.

Growing up, I was surrounded by old people. Over forty was considered *old*. Talking to people in their seventies and eighties was a daily event. People were made of tough stuff in the anthracite region of northeastern Pennsylvania; the older generation was tough and uncompromising. They didn't tolerate nonsense—from kids or anyone else. If you crossed the line (real or imagined), you'd get a sharp tongue-lashing. If words didn't do the job, they might just throw whatever was within reach.

Respecting seniors wasn't a suggestion. It was a deeply held cultural value. Elders were considered wise, worthy of deference. They were our connection to the past, and they carried hard-earned knowledge that demanded respect. This was distinctly American. We were told...

"Respect your elders."

"Be nice to old people."

"Age and experience bring wisdom."

"Old people are our link to history."

But today, that's changed. Now, older people are often dismissed as irrelevant or inconvenient. Google and AI have replaced lived experience. Young and middle-aged people view older people as obstacles to their success—or a complete pain in the ass.

You see this casual disregard everywhere today, in the workplace, on the street, in stores.

For healthy independent older adults living on their own terms, this disrespect is simply background noise. A transient indignity. But this chapter isn't about the older adults who still live on their own terms.

It's about those who can't, and the behaviors that tell the real story—actions that contradict the polite words we use when we talk about how we "honor" our elders.

Because when you watch what they do, what becomes clear is this: Disrespect for nursing home residents isn't just common.

It's an open secret.

The Helping Handout of Medicaid

Imagine it's election season. Immaculately dressed and coiffed candidates campaigning. Big smiles, firm handshakes, and booming voices on every channel and commercial break.

In debates, sound bites, or full-throated rhetoric, you'll hear these talking points driven through their messaging:

"I will be a voice for seniors!"

"I will protect our poor and disenfranchised!"

"I won't rest until the job is done!"

These words. Said every year, or two, or four.

One subject routinely avoided—on the campaign trail and elsewhere—are the financial hardships most nursing home patients endure, specifically those receiving Medicaid, the payor covering the majority of the nation's nursing home population.

For the individual nursing home patient, achieving Medicaid eligibility requires near destitution, as states have maximum asset allowances.

With few exceptions, Medicaid's individual asset maximum is $2,000.

Consider that. You're sick and down to your last two grand.

Once Medicaid-approved, a nursing home patient relinquishes control of their monthly income from pension or Social Security. In return for receiving Medicaid nursing home benefits, the income previously received now becomes part of the formula by which the home is paid.

For example, suppose a person—while living in their community—receiving $1,000 monthly in Social Security income now requires nursing home care. Once transferred to the nursing home and approved for Medicaid, this $1,000 monthly income is now treated like this:

- The patient receives a portion of this $1,000 income in the form of a Personal Needs Allowance (PNA). Allowance levels are determined by each state.
- The nursing home receives the remainder of the patient's income.
- The nursing home bills the state Medicaid program for the balance of the patient's care not covered by the patient's income.

A patient's PNA is the *maximum* amount of monthly income a patient receives to spend on items *not* provided by the nursing home. Said differently, this is the money that a state lets a patient have for personal enjoyment—to enhance their quality of life.

Here's a short list of items nursing homes don't provide that a PNA might be used for:

- Clothes
- Shoes
- Socks and underwear
- Makeup and perfume
- A haircut

- A television
- A phone
- A Hershey Bar
- A gift for a loved one
- A pack of Marlboros

So, what's a patient's allowance for these things?

I frequently visit The ABC's of Long Term Care Insurance (https://gotltci.com/phyllis-shelton/.), a site providing practical, state-specific information on insurance and long-term care.

This is where President of Got LTCi Phyllis Shelton's research on the nursing home patient PNA amounts for each of the fifty states is invaluable. A quick look indicates that Alabama ($30) and California ($35) are at the lower end of the spectrum. Conversely, Florida ($160) and Alaska ($200) are among the highest in monthly PNAs for Medicaid patients.[4]

For reference, as part of the Omnibus Budget Reconciliation Act of 1987 (OBRA-87), which became effective on July 1, 1988, the PNA was mandated to be increased from $25 to $30 in all states.[5]

This was almost *forty years ago*.

Over this same period, courtesy of AARP's Social Security Resource Center, Americans have received a Social Security Cost-of-Living-Adjustment (COLA) in every year except 2009, 2010, and 2015.[6]

And yet, there's no requirement to apply a COLA to a nursing home patient's PNA.

In the 1750s—forever and ever ago—Jean-Jacques Rousseau's said something very close to, "Money can't buy happiness."[7] Conversely, Gertrude Stein is credited with saying, "Whoever said money can't buy happiness simply didn't know where to go shopping."[8]

Decide for yourself whether Rousseau or Stein is right. Adjusting the 1988 federally-mandated $30 monthly PNA for inflation brings it to an absurdly low $70 today, a level at which several states remain woefully short.

As a result, nursing home patients can't afford some simple pleasures on these monthly allowances. Certainly not without a lot of help.

Try this at home ... find your state's monthly Medicaid PNA amount. See how far this amount goes in covering the daily or weekly pleasures *you* enjoy today.

I did, and didn't do too well. How about you?

One last item to know about Medicaid recipients and their monthly PNAs is that not every patient receives their income on time—or at all.

Why?

Patients who coordinate deposit of their Social Security check with the nursing home have little difficulty in receiving their monthly income. Accounting approaches and applications ensure the nursing home is paid and the patient income is provided on schedule.

Alternatively, when patients (or their representatives) don't coordinate payment and receipt of patient income, delays are likely for home and patient. Family members sometimes opt to control banking and financial management on a patient's behalf, creating risks of this money being diverted for other purposes.

Unfortunately, these behaviors have resulted in the nursing home not being paid the patient's monthly share of cost under Medicaid—and the patient never seeing their PNA.

Charity helps fill gaps created by monthly PNA shortfalls and social dysfunction. Coat drives, new socks and underwear donations, and community organizations offering the gift of time and attention are difference-makers.

Some organizations bring Christmas to nursing homes—including food and gifts for every patient—every single year. Nursing home employees make cash or in-kind contributions, as do families, sometimes with significant posthumous gifts.

Still, these efforts leave patients with wardrobes consisting largely of string-tied hospital gowns and foot covers, and others which take on the daily appearance of a Second Hand Rose or Joe the Rag Man.

So the next time you hear candidates bellowing, "I will protect our poor and disenfranchised!" look beyond their words and at their behaviors directed to the nursing home patients they are representing.

The COVID Double Standard

A nursing home isn't a flower shop. Never has been. Never will be.

Caring for sick people can be very scary. Plenty of ink has been devoted to the coronavirus over the past few years, and yet COVID isn't the only health risk to nursing home patients.

Nursing home patients will catch colds, if not from other patients, from caregivers or visitors. Even with vaccinations, there will be occasions when the flu strikes. An upper respiratory or gastrointestinal infection could make patients wish they'd never entered a home.

Other health risks—that may be lesser known—can't be discounted. Antibiotic resistant infections, including methicillin-resistant Staphylococcus aureus (MRSA) and vancomycin-resistant enterococci (VRE) are two that dominate caregiver attention when present in patients.

This *alphabet soup* of illnesses sends workers to the exits, and patients to the hospital or a premature death. One thing to remember, though. These same illnesses or infections can be acquired:

- Vacationing on a cruise ship
- Attending a sporting event
- Dining in a restaurant
- Attending a class
- Coming together for a holiday
- Going through airport security

Nurses and certified nursing assistants—with the help of physicians, infection control specialists, and pharmacists—display great skill in treating and controlling the spread of these infections. Many nursing homes are very good at this.

This is the environmental landscape. It has been for decades. Some people recover from these illnesses and infections. Others don't.

In early 2020, COVID changed this landscape, and quite possibly permanently. It might be due to what *one* person said, and the subsequent behaviors of *many*.

On March 10, 2020, in the pandemic's early days and at what might have been the height of attention for the Life Care Center of Kirkland, Washington, during its designation as Ground Zero, American Health Care Association (AHCA) President Mark Parkinson appeared on CNN's *At This Hour* with Kate Bolduan.[9]

After Ms. Bolduan teed up the topic, Mr. Parkinson responded with this as his first sentence:

"The grim reality is that for the elderly, COVID-19 is almost a perfect killing machine."

This sentence scared, shocked, and horrified nursing home patients, family members, and workers—across the nation.

As a result, one has to believe that people stopped listening and started drawing their own conclusions.

ᔓ

The reality is that on March 10, 2020, it was very, very, early, and there were many, many more unknowns than knowns.

As the interview continued, Mr. Parkinson made additional statements on the industry's behalf:

- "We are dealing with perhaps the greatest challenge that we have ever had in the history of our sector."
- "We are encouraging all people, including family members

and loved ones, to not visit nursing homes and assisted living facilities."

- "Our guidance as of today is to family members, to loved ones, don't visit the facilities."
- "We want you to be in constant contact with your loved one, we just don't want you in the buildings, possibly spreading the virus."

As a nursing home executive, I recall the conflict created by this messaging. If this virus truly was a perfect killing machine for the elderly, risks were incredibly high that a loved one might die while in the nursing home and not be seen again by their loved ones living in the community.

Tragically, this posture violated one of the decades-old reasons for placing people into nursing homes—a solution to loneliness.

As a patient's son, the indifference to a patient's quality of life and maintaining continuity with friends and family was overpowering.

Because what I heard was—*It's no longer safe for you to go see someone that you love.*

These talking points, from a trade association executive rather than a state or federal lawmaker, resulted in an immediate, nationwide restriction to long-standing regulations allowing nursing home patients the right to receive visitors.

And at the time of these statements, it would be months before nursing homes in many states received their first—alleged or confirmed—COVID-positive patient.

Near the interview's conclusion, Ms. Bolduan inquired about families who no longer trusted nursing homes to care of their loved one and wanted to take them home. Responding, Mr. Parkinson strongly encouraged families not to take people out of nursing homes, due to the risks associated with transfer trauma and acquiring the virus in the community.

To nursing home administrators, patients, and families, this meant, *It also isn't safe for your loved one to come see you.*

This double-edged guidance—visitors shouldn't come into, and patients shouldn't come out of a nursing home—coupled with the "perfect killing machine" moniker left people searching for answers.

Based on his guidance—no visitors in, or patients out—Mr. Parkinson implied that the community *was* the COVID risk factor for nursing home patients. Yet as nursing homes were labeled as Ground Zero for the virus, workers were leaving their homes—in communities—each day, to care for these same patients.

Mixed message? Double standard? You decide. One question that remains, over five years later: *Was anyone asking patients what they wanted?*

Lasting Consequences

Mark Parkinson's words couldn't be unheard.

Among working seniors, the sentiments *I don't want to* or *My body or soul won't let me* became the new post-COVID normal. Based on October 2022 estimates provided by the US Federal Reserve Board, "the retired share of the US population was nearly 1½ percentage points above its pre-pandemic level ... accounting for nearly all of the shortfall in the labor force participation rate." [10]

One and one-half percent might not seem like a large gap, until it's applied to approximately 170 million US workers. Then, it equals 2,550,000 people.

For some older nursing home workers, the challenges of patient care exceeded their intention of serving others.

Why? People got scared and went away. Their person-specific fears included:

- *I might get sick.*
- *My family might get sick.*
- *I might die.*

In nursing homes, these risks have been true for decades. Nevertheless, COVID appears to be the seminal event that turned the world inside out for their workers. I believe this happened because people became scared of nursing homes and their patients. An unintended consequence of what one person said, and the subsequent behaviors of many.

Today, nursing homes are still hurting badly. Their outcry is that staffing is a problem of epic proportions. And it is.

COVID laid bare a weakness that might be unable to be converted to a strength. Left unabated, it's an existential threat to nursing homes.

Will it cause the industry's death? I don't think so. There are nursing homes and companies today that are strong, stable, and growing. They'll survive and prosper. I do, however, think that in the aftermath of what transpired, a very different landscape will emerge.

Let's look at the staffing issues since the pandemic.

In November 2021, AHCA—based on statistics released by the Bureau of Labor Statistics, covering the period March 2020 through October 2021—stated that 221,000 workers (or 14 percent of its workforce) left the nursing homes.[11]

This is what people getting scared and going away looks like.

In May 2022, a *Skilled Nursing News* article, "No Magic Bullet: How Operators are Rethinking Their Staffing Strategies," estimated "more than 400,000 caregivers have exited the industry since the start of the pandemic (source not cited)."[12]

This is what more people getting scared and going away looks like. Or the result of worker fatigue from covering those leaving in the initial exodus.

By January 2023, almost three years following COVID's nursing home presence, AHCA, in their *Long-Term Care Jobs Report*, reported worker deficit at 210,000. Additionally, they indicated that "all long-term care employees at a thirteen-year low" and that "long-term care: worst impacted than any other health care sector."[13]

Comparatively, this report highlights nursing homes as experiencing the largest workforce destruction in the healthcare sector. This grid highlights the changes:

EMPLOYMENT CHANGE—FEBRUARY 2020 - DECEMBER 2022			
Sector	**Number of Jobs**	**Gained/ Lost**	**Workforce Change**
Physician Offices	157,700	Gained	+5.8%
Outpatient Care	42,100	Gained	+4.2%
Home Health	55,300	Gained	+3.6%
Hospitals	43,700	Gained	+0.8%
Assisted Living	4,200	Lost	-.0.9%
Nursing Homes	**210,000**	**Lost**	**-13.3%**

Aside from assisted living, which reported a less than 1 percent workforce loss, other segments responsible for providing direct care to Americans grew and prospered, rebounding fully and then some. This is good news. Unless you're in the nursing home business.

While these sectors differ, they each share these common themes:

- The work is hard.
- It involves taking care of people who are sick or hurt.

So after billions in Paycheck Protection Program (PPP), Coronavirus Aid, Relief, and Economic Security (CARES) Act, and state Medicaid money was appropriated to nursing homes, resulting in enhancements to workforce compensation programs like special pay, hero pay, retention pay, COVID unit pay, and increases in starting pay, nursing home workers voted with their feet and didn't come back. I believe this continues because people remain scared of nursing homes and their patients.

ᘓ

Workforce distress extends beyond a nursing home's four walls, or a management company's organizational chart. Many states have experienced extraordinary difficulties in their own staffing, specifically for nursing home surveyors. When this happens, states will find it nearly impossible to survey each nursing home within the nine-to-fifteen month period required by the Centers for Medicare and Medicaid Services (CMS) and effectively investigate complaint allegations regarding patient care, patient rights, and compliance.

In a July 2023 *Skilled Nursing News* article, "Strained by Survey Challenges, Nursing Home Operators Cite Inexperienced Inspection Teams," hardships in survey staffing were cited in the following states:[14]

- Kentucky, where less than one in five surveyor positions were filled as of October 2022.
- Minnesota, whose agency's federal survey team vacancy rate was 30 percent, and became 25 percent.
- North Carolina, with 420 nursing homes, fewer than 100 inspectors, a 15 percent vacancy rate, and nearly 35 percent annual turnover.
- West Virginia, where 44 percent of (surveyor) positions were currently vacant.

Just over a week later, this publication, in "Staffing Shortages Cause Survey Backlog for Half of Connecticut Skilled Nursing Facilities, in Tandem With More Immediate Jeopardy Cases," put surveyor vacancy rates between 20 percent and 25 percent, compared to 40 percent just a year prior.[15]

This short list encompasses several states, affecting more than a thousand nursing homes. In March 2024, however, the US Senate Special

Committee on Aging released a national view of state surveyor vacancies in its special report—*Uninspected and Neglected*.[16] For those interested in learning substantially more about state and federal oversight of the nation's nursing homes, this report is invaluable.

Buried in the appendices of this report is a table highlighting state surveyor vacancy, comparing 2002 and 2022. This grid illustrates a sample of state-specific performance:[17]

STATE SURVEYOR VACANCIES 2002 VS. 2022		
State	**2002**	**2022**
Alabama	10%	80%
Arkansas	20%	40%
Indiana	18%	1%
New Jersey	23%	53%
Ohio	5%	25%
Oklahoma	4%	45%
Texas	20%	13%
Virginia	5%	31%

Surprising? Yes. Unfortunately, this problem continues today.

From various sources, states continue to experience surveyor staffing deficiencies, with unmanaged backlogs in survey and critical follow-up on patient-related issues.

- Kansas, where only twenty-nine of sixty-one surveyor positions—dedicated to investigating between 7,000 and 9,000 annual complaints of abuse, neglect, and exploitation—are filled.[18]
- New York, where 120 of 163 nursing homes in the city's five boroughs *haven't* been inspected in the past fifteen months, and thirty-three haven't been inspected since 2021.[19]

Other states and stories are out there. It's apparent that this issue isn't isolated to the homes, and includes those agencies paid to keep an eye on them.

Growing up, and for decades after, employment with the state or the government or in civil service was very highly sought. Predictable work, job security, weekends off, pension plans, and representation at the bargaining table were main attractions.

I still believe that these reasons apply. Just not for nursing home surveyor positions, right now.

Why? Hard to know. A root cause analysis on this would be purely speculative. So, let's speculate a little.

- People got used to their new lifestyles during COVID. Surveyors too. As a result, some opted for early retirement. As of April 2023, economic research done by The Federal Reserve Bank of St. Louis estimated "approximately 2.4 million excess retirees in the US ... still well above our predicted trend."[20]
- People may have sought and received transfers within their state's employment system, nurses in particular.
- It is possible, though highly unlikely, that many workers transferred to the private sector, lured by juicy sign-on bonuses and a bigger payday.

Surveyors are everyday people, just like nursing home workers. The words they heard couldn't be unheard, and their concerns couldn't be promised away by their employers. As a result, they left and haven't returned.

I believe this happened because people became scared, and remain scared of nursing homes and their patients.

And as a result, states examined the cost to restore their workforces—in competitive wages, benefits, and working conditions, with many deciding to outsource these oversight tasks to nongovernmental, third-party organizations—at increased costs—rather than grappling with the challenges of recruiting, training, and retaining these workers.

Mission Reversal and Market Confusion

Preparing for this work, I reviewed numerous industry publications supporting the narratives that the industry hoped to sear into the public's consciousness. Among many, one emerged as *the* refrain of owners and leaders:

The importance of their company's culture.

Culture—plus more money and people—were the solution to all problems.

In the midst and aftermath of COVID, as nursing home companies benefited from massive taxpayer funding and relaxed regulation, this cultural mantra became known as:

"Residents Second."

Confused? I was. Especially after reading the October 10, 2022 *Skilled Nursing News* article "Why AHCA's Parkinson Predicts a Nursing Home Sector Recovery—and How to Get There," which recounted remarks made by Mark Parkinson during the of AHCA/National Center for Assisted Living (NCAL) 2022 annual convention.[21]

During the opening general session, Mr. Parkinson is quoted as stating:

"These companies and buildings that are doing great have great leaders who are committed to developing ... In fact many of them tell me that patients and *residents come second* because employees come first." (emphasis added)

Their rationale: Because workers *create the experience* for nursing home patients, the shift among nursing homes is to put *employees first*, and patients (or residents) second.

Plausible? Maybe. But ... for a nursing home?

Their supporting argument was that without employees—more importantly, happy employees—delivering a positive patient experience was not possible.

Here's the part that isn't receiving as much attention. They were short workers and it is incredibly hard to get them back.

Something had to be done.

After workers exited—deciding there weren't enough reasons to return—it is curious that these two words, *Residents Second,* were selected—by nursing home owners and executives—to describe the desired culture they intended to create.

Sticking with this notion for a moment, let's examine a few business types, testing a thesis similar to "residents second."

- Welcome to Horace Mann Elementary. Our Motto: *Teachers first, Students second!*
- "I'm sorry that you ordered prime rib. The cook made grilled cheese, and we are an *employee-first* business."
- "I've credited your account with $1,000, rather than $2,000 from this deposit. It might be a mistake, *but our employer tells us that the employees are always right."*

These extremes are shared to illustrate the mission and market confusion resulting from the intentional shifts away from those intended to receive services.

As a practical matter, nursing homes are defenseless when challenged over this public posture of "residents second."

There's no nuance here. Strictly speaking, these statements, in published interviews, marketing materials, or intercompany communication, are contrary to a nursing home's mission.

Additionally, the pleas of industry trade association representatives, lobbyists, and company executives are totally neutralized when seeking additional taxpayer funding from Medicare or Medicaid programs.

Finally, this ordinal ranking—by a home, company, or industry—placing workers above those receiving care will result in patients, families, advocates, and others asking:

If *my resident* is first to me, why are they second to you?

ꟹ

Life isn't simple for a nursing home. Workers, as free agents, can choose to work anywhere they're in demand. When choosing a nursing home, it's because they're willing to do the hard work of taking care of people who are unable to take care of themselves.

Among their many goals is providing dignified care to those patients while recognizing and respecting their needs. A concurrent goal is to work in a reciprocal environment, where their efforts are respected and treated with dignity—by their direct supervisor, the home's leadership, and the home's ownership.

Improving an individual home or company culture is laudable. I'd argue, however, the industrial mantra of "residents second," even for a limited duration, doesn't help achieve this. It's one thing to say "workers first," but the industry really went wrong with taking that concept one step further and actively promoting this alternative slogan. Disrespect for the patient is painfully evident when these words are written ... and said.

Something attributed to the late NASCAR superstar Dale Earnhardt may provide clarity around "residents second." His famous and oft-repeated quote is especially germane here. "Second place is first loser."

Great nursing homes know this, and put *people*—patients and workers, both—*first.*

WHAT YOU CAN DO

Ask Questions About:

- The COVID experience, lessons learned and changes made since 2020.
- Techniques to maintain connections between people.
- Workforce changes, including people lost, gained, and replaced with agency or third-parties.
- Survey frequency since 2021, and state agency (Department of Health or equivalent) responsiveness to complaints received.

Look for:

- Public messaging about People. What's written, by whom, and for what purpose?
- Behaviors … are they consistent with what's been said or written?
- Published information about surveyor staffing deficiencies, health department funding, and delays in investigating abuse, neglect, or exploitation?

Listen to What People Say:

- Can you identify their priority?
- Does it sound like there's alignment between priorities and mission?

III

THE TRUTH HAS BEEN EASY TO HIDE

True or False: The sun rises in the east and sets in the west.

Answer: Both true and false.

Scientists have concluded that the sun rises *exactly* in the east—and sets *exactly* in the west—two days a year, making "True" a correct answer.

Conversely, the remainder of the year, the sun rises *generally* in the east, and sets *generally* in the west, making "False" a correct answer.

Or would it? Depends on your application. In the strictest sense, "Both" seems to apply, making the truth very hard to find.

Truths—important ones—can hide in plain sight. Like a game of Telephone, or long-standing urban myths, statements which aren't true, generally or specifically, become regarded as fact.

Indisputable, incontrovertible, unassailable facts.

This chapter addresses some of these beliefs. If it doesn't fully convert myths to facts, it may—in the end—provide a different definition of the truth.

Myth #1—Healthcare Has Two Tiers

Attending my very first lecture in business school, an exceptionally well-dressed, eloquent, white-haired health economist prepared to dazzle an assembly of graduate students on the state of US healthcare.

For ninety minutes, he pounded the existence of *two-tiered* healthcare, in which a subset of Americans received healthcare from:

- Public programs financed with taxpayer dollars
- Programs financed privately, with premiums paid by individuals or their employers

This was the prevailing belief in 1984 as explained in this lecture hall, and continues to be embraced today.

Consistently, this healthcare economist, and others over the next forty years, insisted that the tiers within US healthcare were:

Two.

I think this is total BS. And hiding in plain sight.

Grouping payor sources, such as governmental payors like Medicaid, and all other payor sources, has resulted in the narrative—like my ol' professor said—of a "two-tiered" healthcare system.

I believe, based on decades of observation and experience, there are at least *seven* tiers linked to nursing home care, based on the insurance plan or person responsible for payment. These include:

- Private insurance
- Private pay (cash)
- Medicare
- Medicare Advantage
- Managed care
- Medical assistance (Medicaid)
- Veterans Administration (VA)

Two tiers? Not even close.

To working colleagues who rarely saw, touched, or communicated with nursing home patients, I routinely shared two thoughts:

- A nursing home's job—when possible—is to help patients improve, with returning home as a goal.
- When a person returns home, it's impractical to believe that they will be good as new.

Instead, a person is likely a different version of "whole," and not the same before the event causing their hospitalization and nursing home admission.

At discharge, a person may fully resemble themselves prior to their event. Once home, it's important that the person—now a *former* patient—is able to do their best work, enjoying their best possible life in this different version of their whole self.

Nursing homes incorporating this philosophy into discussing, examining, and caring for patients create environments ripe for success.

ꕤ

No two patients are alike—in their care needs *or* insurance benefits. Payments to nursing homes also differ by a patient's insurance plan.

There's a temptation to classify anything that has "Medi_ _ _ _" in its name, and group into a single tier. Then, add VA, and define all as taxpayer-funded, governmental administered, third-party insurers.

Nursing homes are wise when resisting this temptation. Otherwise, a home's business model may be short-lived, threatening its continued existence, and in the process—harming patients.

Each tier is materially different, by underlying funding source, the percentage contributed, and rules, including patient coverage and eligibility guidelines. They differ administratively, including program oversight. Industry sentiment for patients within these tiers depends on payor behavior, participation requirements, and amounts reimbursed for care.

Unsurprisingly, private insurance and privately-paying patients are the most highly sought, as they allow a home to bypass administrative or bureaucratic hurdles associated with other payors, especially when paying by cash or credit card.

The hardship for nursing homes is that *few* patients fall within these tiers. People with this financial leverage will pursue home and community-based options before a nursing home.

Beneficiaries of long-term care insurance, for example, explore every available option to use what their plan provides to receive care in their home or at another location.

My own long-term care insurance policy allows for its monthly benefit to be used with provider(s) I choose to help meet my own care needs.

While annual premiums for this insurance can be a disqualifier, I have no regrets having purchased this coverage at age forty. My plan will be paid in full at age sixty-five, with annual inflation escalators for the plan's duration, helping to offset increases in the cost of care as I get older or my needs increase.

My wife's long-term care insurance plan is fully paid, with features identical to mine, and no continuing costs to carry. If you ever have the inclination to consider this coverage for yourself, it's worth a look, considering all of life's possibilities before deciding. We did and have enjoyed the accompanying peace of mind ever since.

People paying with cash also have incredible agility in designing a personalized, noninstitutional approach to their care. I've known privately-paying patients who opted for a nursing home to escape the hovering of family members or simply for some peace and quiet during a time when they needed care.

Some eventually returned home, while others created their own personal oasis, remaining for their life's duration. As my career progressed, patients in the latter category were an anomaly, due to the variety of home and community-based services and the proliferation of world-class assisted living offerings.

A brief aside—during the 1990s, as an alternative to nursing home and assisted living placement, seniors with cash (or income) opted instead to receive their care aboard ... *cruise ships.* This trend is enjoying a renaissance, and is indicative of what people possessing the freedom to choose will ... choose!

Here's a sampling of headlines specific to this movement:

- Couple booked fifty-one back-to-back cruises instead of retiring to a nursing home.[22]
- Could "Golden Passport" tempt older adults to swap senior living for cruise ship living?[23]

Pictures of the couple opting for fifty-one cruises showed happy, smiling people. And preliminary research of the Golden Passport, offered by Villa Vie Residences, indicates pricing, services, accommodations, and itineraries well suited to stimulate conversations for people with interest—*and options.*[24]

At the extreme opposite of the tiers are people whose insurance program is the payor of last resort. While earlier chapters have touched on Medicaid and the associated travails of nursing home patients, there are tiers within this payor-based tier bearing exploration.

For this tier alone, nursing home workers must understand and navigate coverage, eligibility, and risk associated with patients in the following Medicaid-related designations:

- Short-Term Private, converting to Medicaid Pending (paying cash until meeting eligibility for Medicaid program participation)
- Medicaid Pending (awaiting program approval)
- Dually-Eligible Medicaid (also receiving Medicare benefits)
- Dually-Eligible Medicaid w/o Medicare Part B
- Managed Medicaid (a third-party, nonstate agency administers coverage, eligibility, provider contracting/credentialing, and payment)

Though complex, this is what a nursing home faces in decisions involving program participation, patient evaluation, patient selection, coordination of benefits, interactions with families and responsible parties, and physician coverage.

Two tiers? No way.

Casting additional light on Medicaid's "tiers within a tier," one thing more bears comment. Though easier, it's less accurate (and more risky) for a nursing home to classify candidates for admission or patients—once admitted—as either a Short-Term Private converting to Medicaid or Medicaid Pending.

Why? Because like a place-kicked football approaching the crossbar and lined up between the goal posts cannot be deemed GOOD until it successfully *clears the other side* of the crossbar, an applicant for Medicaid cannot be deemed a beneficiary until they are *approved* for insurance coverage.

Until the applicant is approved for Medicaid coverage, they're in an entirely different tier. Duration until approval can be unpredictable. As a result, these patients—in the absence of another taxpayer-funded primary payor—should be viewed as paying privately.

These situations present challenging times for administrators. Collecting payments due and receiving cooperation of all parties central to successfully filing and completing the Medicaid application process can be all-consuming.

VA beneficiaries aren't immune to navigating multiple tiers for nursing home care. The majority of the nation's veterans experience similar requirements for age, income, net worth, coverage, eligibility, and payment as others, falling into one of the tiers previously covered.

Based on thresholds for each of these variables, veterans may qualify for a VA pension to help offset the cost of skilled nursing. Visit www.va.gov for specifics.

In other situations, veterans may qualify for short or long-term stays in a community-based nursing home, providing the home meets criteria specifically outlined by the VA. In many states, the VA surveys its contracted nursing homes separately, issuing their own statement of deficiencies and requiring a plan of correction.

Specific workforce hurdles must be cleared for a nursing home to contract with the VA, including prevailing wage rates and fringe benefit packages. Nursing homes in communities with low expectations of patient volume won't pursue a VA provider agreement due to unfavorable cost/benefit calculations of revenues expected versus costs of maintaining contract eligibility.

Last, based on eligibility criteria, veterans may receive skilled nursing care in a State Veterans Home. These nursing homes are owned by state governments, paid by the VA, and often operated under a third-party management contract with another skilled nursing management company.

From the VA's website, "Each state establishes eligibility and admission criteria for its homes, and some State Veterans Homes may admit non-Veteran spouses and gold star parents."[25]

Maybe I was wrong. Sorting through all the tiers within tiers, it looks like there are more than *seven* tiers of healthcare within the nursing home business.

ꞩ

No two patients are alike—in their care needs *or* insurance benefits. However, the standard for care most definitely is. For the nursing home, payor status is not a determinant of the care—or services—that a patient is entitled to receive. While the approach to care will differ by person, what the patient has a right to receive doesn't.

If you're inclined to check it out, www.cms.gov, or 42 Code of Federal Regulations, Section 483,[26] provides the behavior and performance expectations of nursing homes.

Alternatively, California Advocates for Nursing Home Reform

(CANHR) does a fine job aggregating content from these sources, articulating the standard to which homes are held for every patient.

"[Nursing homes] are required to help each resident attain or maintain the highest practicable physical, mental, and psychosocial well-being. Care, treatment and therapies must be used to maintain and improve health to the extent possible, subject to the resident's right to choose and refuse services. Unless it is medically unavoidable, nursing homes must ensure that a resident's condition does not decline."[27]

You see, once a nursing home commits to admitting a patient, they *own* the responsibility of caring for the patient. The whole patient. Everything about the patient.

No shortcuts or excuses to be laid at the feet of an insurance plan beneficiary, their coverage, or their eligibility. *Payor sources and tiers be damned.* In CANHR's synopsis, nothing remotely mentions tier, payor, insurance company, or case manager.

So for all the rhetoric surrounding two-tiered healthcare, and the contrarian information shared thus far, it's important to know that **there is only one standard.**

And according to this standard, **all patients are to be treated equally**. And it's the nursing home's job to figure out exactly how this is to be done.

Myth #2—Medicare and Medicare Advantage Are a Lot Alike

Having covered the extremes among tiers, we'll examine those that nursing homes—and their owners and executives—pursue with obsession.

These include Medicare—or by beneficiary election, Medicare Advantage—and Managed Care. We'll begin by separating these taxpayer-funded, government-administered tiers into their parts.

Among nursing home leaders, Medicare is considered *the industry's salvation,* as the average daily revenue a home receives per patient ranks highest among other payors and tiers.

A strong and stable source of Medicare revenue offsets any losses associated with patients in other tiers, such as Medicaid.

Within companies, Medicare patient population (or mix) is often considered the singular predictive indicator of a nursing home's market strength. Homes with the highest Medicare mix—even for a moment in time—will receive greater praise and respect from executives, and a level of respect that may (or may not) be justly due.

Poll veteran nursing home executives for their favorite stories of annual budgeting or acquisition due diligence, and you'll hear tales of owners and senior executives extolling the strategic advantages of additional Medicare business.

My favorite was during acquisition due diligence of an underperforming nursing home. The company's brain trust—the CEO and other equity partners, while reviewing the home's history and proposed financial statements, chattered:

"You know, if we can increase census 9-10 Medicare (patients per day), we are golden."

Like the fable of the goose and her eggs. Golden.

Most importantly, Medicare patients serve as the fuel for related-party ancillary businesses, a force multiplier for owners of rehabilitation services, pharmacy, dialysis, and other companies which can generate substantial profits without the financial disclosure requirements of nursing homes.

We'll deeply explore this dimension in the next chapter.

ꕤ

Medicare Advantage—defined here as *Medicare's cousin*—shares common elements with Medicare, though a closer look indicates something completely different.

Participation requires the beneficiary to sign up for Medicare Parts A and B, then *trade-in* their Medicare benefits for a Medicare Advantage plan.[28]

Medicare Advantage occasionally comes with a celebrity twist. These are the insurance plans where 1960s and 1970s icons such as Joe Namath, Jimmie "JJ" Walker, and William Shatner on TV commercials hawk the features and benefits of plans and the call centers that will help them *get started.*

Yes, Broadway Joe, J. J. Evans, and Captain James T. Kirk are paid to convince people to dump coverage with Uncle Sam and call 1-800-YABBA-DABBA-DOO.

And people do it.

In return, people receive hospital and physician coverage, similar to Medicare Parts A and B. They also receive coverage for prescription medications. Plans may offer other benefits like dental, vision, transportation, fitness center membership, or home-delivered meals.

Receiving these benefits are subject to rules set by the insurance company administering the Medicare Advantage plan. Your hospital, physicians, and nursing homes must participate within the plan's limited provider network. Out-of-state providers are frequently out-of-bounds for beneficiaries, which is distinctly *different* from Medicare.[29]

Additional out-of-pocket costs may apply for certain services, requiring a careful look before choosing. In some markets, there are numerous plans available—with features, benefits, and cost sharing requirements that will leave people age 65 and older downright dizzy.

Using statistics from the Kaiser Family Foundation (KFF),[30] the average Medicare beneficiary had over forty Medicare Advantage plans to choose from. By contrast, Medicare is a singular plan, with its only option administered by Uncle Sam.

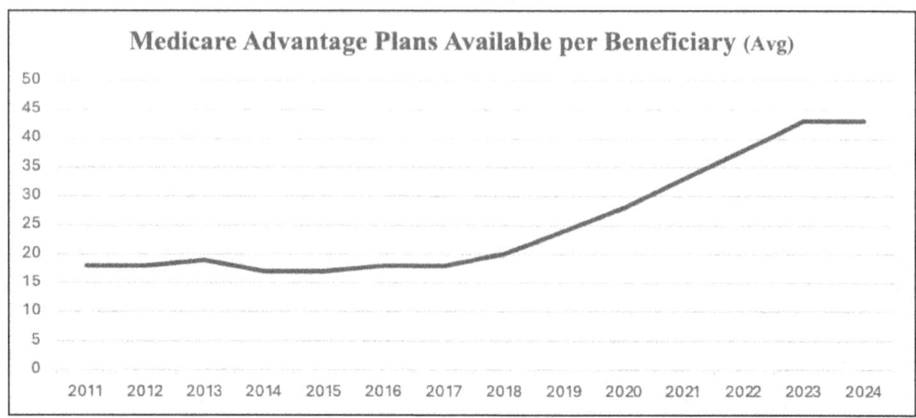

One final element separating Medicare Advantage from Medicare is the role of the primary care physician, who serves as gatekeeper on behalf of the beneficiary and is the first in a line of many decision-makers paid to actively *manage the care* a person receives.

In this *managed care* approach, attention is incessant, regarding care by:

- Type
- Amount
- Cost

Historically favored by nursing home leaders and their salesforces, Medicare Advantage provided two things attractive to decision-makers—*scale, and something that wasn't Medicaid.*

Here's an illustration of scale:

By the end of 2024, 54 percent of Medicare-eligible beneficiaries, or thirty-three million people, had enrolled in a Medicare Advantage program.[31]

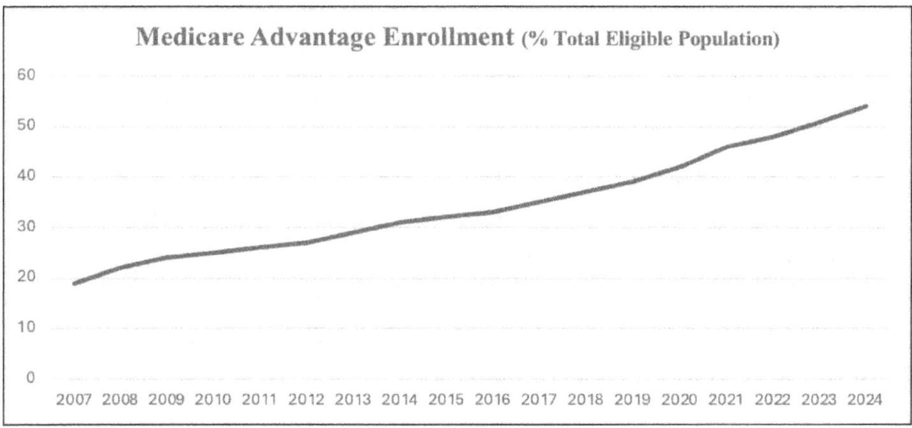

These numbers are tough to ignore. They didn't occur accidentally either.

If you've not been to a Medicare Advantage enrollment ***party*** presentation at a senior center, private home, local restaurant, or hotel conference room, this is what the experience might be:

An attractive, well-dressed, and eloquent Medicare account representative (or similar title) associated with a health plan hosts a gathering for sixty-somethings seeking to learn more about Medicare.

The route taken in securing attendees' undivided attention? Food. Pastry, fruit, juice, coffee.

Good coffee.

Sales approaches—expertly delivered by mature, confident women, engendering trust among attendees—might include touting preventive care at *zero* dollars (just like Medicare), a 24/7 nurse help line, eyeglasses, transportation, and SilverSneakers.

What's SilverSneakers? "Available at no cost for adults sixty-five and older through select *Medicare plans*. Senior fitness programs to help you stay active and feel great." (emphasis included).[32]

Whoa! OK, how does this stack up with information straight from Medicare's own website (www.medicare.org)? Specific to the question,

"Does Original Medicare cover SilverSneakers?" Medicare's response is, "Original Medicare, Part A and B, does not cover this benefit."[33]

Confusing? Yes. SilverSneakers hasn't always included the word *Advantage*.

Increasingly, whether it's the gym membership, the transportation, or the 24/7 help line, people are buying what these incredibly sharp and seemingly trustworthy Medicare account representatives are selling.

Why? This is the closer, from Better Medicare Alliance in May 2021:

"96 percent of Medicare Advantage beneficiaries have access to at least one zero-dollar premium plan"[34]

Zero. And Americans love a giveaway!

So ... they grab a pen and choose Blue Cross Blue Shield, Aetna, UnitedHealthcare, and others as their Medicare Advantage health plan.

Numbers confirm this behavior. As of November 2023, 84 percent of beneficiaries chose zero-premium plans for the 2023 coverage year; for 2022 that figure was 88 percent.[35]

While down slightly, year-over-year, 84 percent is a massive number.

My fear, based on experience, is that as times get really rough, beneficiaries might be disappointed in what they get. *Zero*.

As the saying goes—you get *exactly* what you pay for.

Among friends and colleagues, I've referred to this is as *Medicare (Where's the ... ?) Advantage*. Because it's not Medicare, and sometimes I'm searching for the Advantage.

Truth is, Medicare Advantage doesn't exactly follow Medicare guidelines. Though www.medicare.org plainly states, "Medicare Advantage Plans Must Follow CMS Guidelines,"[36] there *must* be some play in the words "follow" or "guidelines."

These plans behave differently than how nursing homes *must* behave when serving patients requiring skilled nursing services.

I'll share two examples:

First, under Medicare Advantage, the qualifying hospital stay requirement is often waived for skilled nursing coverage. I'm intentionally inserting "often" to protect against subsequent surprises, though I've *never* experienced a health plan whose Medicare Advantage program didn't utilize this waiver. Never.

The absence of a three-day qualifying hospital stay—as required by Medicare[37]—allows the health plan to move a patient into a nursing home more rapidly than would otherwise be the case if the patient had Medicare Part A coverage. The less time a patient spends in a hospital means more money saved (and potentially earned) by the health plan.

Does this waiver increase the risk of establishing, or more importantly, maintaining a patient's medical stability? Depends on who one asks.

Second, health plans are parental in case managing a patient's care. Preauthorization and concurrent review routinely occur during a patient's stay, with plans applying their own interpretation of Medicare's skilled coverage guidelines to a patient's condition.

When coverage guidelines are disputed, the health plan prevails. Asking a plan to *quickly* change a coverage decision is very much like asking a pissed-off parent to immediately change their mind about grounding their own child.

It never happens … Never.

Challenging a health plan's unfavorable coverage determination *is* an option for the home and patient. It will be a protracted process, testing the patient's patience and resources, potentially interrupting care continuity and secondary insurance coverage.

If a nursing home strenuously objects to an adverse coverage decision, they risk damaging their contractual relationship with the health plan.

So … they don't do it.

Like squaring off with a parent who punishes without mercy, nursing homes won't risk the institutional fallout of a Medicare Advantage contract being terminated—or patient referral traffic slowed—by righteously advocating on behalf of an individual patient.

By contrast, nursing home decision makers *will* become righteously indignant in defending coverage decisions for patients covered under

Medicare Part A. Those who see, touch, treat, talk with, and listen to their patients *will* take on peers and superiors to allow a patient complete access to their benefits and maintain integrity in administering coverage and eligibility criteria. Additionally, the clock is not a barrier to receiving a rapid response.

These topics never find daylight during a Medicare Advantage enrollment party. People are dazzled with the prospects of *zero* out-of-pocket dollars, SilverSneakers … and the coffee.

Myth #3—Everyone Gets 100 Days

Working with families—thousands—as an administrator and in later roles, cringe-inducing exchanges with those whose loved one was being cared for in a home frequently began with:

"The hospital told me …"

Immediately followed by:

" … everyone gets 100 days."

Once heard, I realized the expectation had been set. A *truth* had been told. It was indisputable, incontrovertible, and unassailable. Mom, Dad, Aunt Bea, or Cousin Eddie would receive 100 days of uninterrupted Medicare coverage in the nursing home—free—if they needed it.

Why*?* Because the hospital said so.

If you've ever been there, and spoken with a hospital discharge planner, case manager, or social worker, about a hospitalized Medicare beneficiary approaching discharge and nursing home placement, you might have heard this. When my mother was hospitalized, a discharge planner told me—point-blank:

"Medicare will pay for your mom's first 100 days in the nursing home."

My experience—dating back to the late 1970s—told me otherwise. The myth, however, was still alive.

This remark is almost rote among hospital workers. Though technically correct, as 100 days is the annual benefit *maximum* for Medicare enrollees,[38] in practicality it's often completely wrong. Patients must satisfy several coverage requirements, including the need for *daily* skilled care as determined by a physician or other healthcare provider. Moreover, if the patient is improving, and the nursing home is doing its job, the likelihood of requiring additional daily skilled care increasingly approaches *zero*.

As a patient's condition improves, the probability of continued coverage under Medicare diminishes. *Yes. Fact.*

In truth, Medicare beneficiaries do receive an annual skilled nursing benefit of 100 days coverage. This benefit's existence, however, doesn't guarantee complete entitlement to exhaust it.

This doesn't keep hospital people from selling the "100 day" line. It sounds good. Good enough for patients to buy it. And when they do, and it doesn't happen—because a patient improves and no longer needs daily skilled care, or their progress stalls or plateaus—they *blame the nursing home, and they blame Medicare.*

Because of this myth and improperly managed expectations, they feel lied to.

The truth, in this case, is very easy to hide.

Deeper within this hidden truth is that during the 100 days that Medicare "pays for," only twenty of these days for skilled nursing coverage will be fully paid by Medicare, meaning the patient incurs *zero* coinsurance liability.

Today, from Day 21 through 100, Medicare patients receiving skilled nursing coverage must pay about $210/day in coinsurance.[39] And it adds up quickly. During these days, while Medicare does pay, they do not pay for everything.

The Day 20/21 timeline is massively disruptive—to homes, patients, and their families. For many patients, the first twenty days' worth of coverage is neither the maximum, nor the optimum, for some Medicare recipients. Patient progress will sometimes exceed this time frame, underscoring the wisdom of the 100-day benefit period.

Nevertheless, patients are prematurely pulled from nursing homes by family members blanching at the prospect of paying the $210 daily coinsurance associated with continued Medicare coverage.

This is further exacerbated in nursing homes unwilling or unable to work with patients and families on a coinsurance repayment plan for the balance of their Medicare stay.

When this traumatic transfer occurs, what is saved—the daily coinsurance payment amount—is too often sacrificed in forfeiting the benefit of patient care continuity. Sadly, I've witnessed this, and have heard similar experiences shared by colleagues over decades.

Today—and likely tomorrow—some patient or family member is going to be told, "Medicare will pay for Cousin Eddie's first 100 days in the nursing home," and this dysfunctional cycle will continue.

Myth #4—Artificial Has Become Better Than Real

Any chapter about Medicare Advantage and nursing homes is incomplete without details of its practical application. Recounting this experience should help.

In the late 2010s, I oversaw a nursing home company whose locations had contracted—for years—with Blue Cross Blue Shield's (BCBS) Medicare Advantage plan. BCBS had recently announced hiring a third-party administrator (TPA) to manage its Medicare Advantage program.

Following BCBS' statewide rollout meetings to providers, I received a copy of their presentation to the nursing home community, "Medicare Advantage Post-Acute Care—Skilled Nursing Facility." It was branded by BCBS and the Blue Care Network of this state, introducing this TPA as their "partner."

I don't know how BCBS paid for this TPA's services (per member per month, percent of shared savings, or an at-risk contracting arrangement), but I'd bet that this new partner was expected to perform utilization management at a cost *cheaper* than BCBS had been able to do it themselves.

The first red flag in reviewing this detail was the TPA's hours of service, 8 a.m.–10 p.m., Monday through Friday, and 10 a.m. to 4 p.m. on holidays and weekends. To some, *this* is comprehensive coverage. Not so much for a business possessing significant leverage over a nursing home. Here's why:

Under its "Expectations," BCBS stated, "Pre-service or prior authorization is obtained—unauthorized transitions should be *rare and justified.*" (emphasis added)

While preauthorization is common with Medicare Advantage and Managed Care plans, "rare" doesn't fit well with businesses like nursing homes and hospitals, which are open and working 24/7. There was zero reference to an on-call line or to late-night or early-weekend service.

One quick aside—for *any* patient admitted to a nursing home before 11:59 p.m., the nursing home can, should, and will count and bill for that calendar day. Just like minutes matter in delivering best possible patient care, they—in this case—matter in delivering best possible business results.

Another key feature of this new partnership was the TPA's predictive functional assessment tool, which would "evaluate more than *260* functional tasks in *20–25* questions," resulting in scores in the areas of Basic Mobility, Daily Activity, and Applied Cognition, as provided in a *predictive outcome* report.

This predictive outcome report could project a number of things, including:

- The amount of time a patient required from a nonskilled caregiver (whatever that is) while in a nursing home
- The amount of time a patient required from a nonskilled caregiver after being discharged to home with home health services

- The anticipated length of stay (in days) in a nursing home
- The projected discharge date from the nursing home
- The therapy cycle while in the nursing home, including the average number of days being treated and the number of minutes per day—based on frequency of treatment—5x, 6x, or 7x/week)

Impressively … fascinating.

BCBS—and their partner—referred to this predictive functional assessment wizard as a "decision-support tool." Curiously, I questioned this tool's purpose.

A) Was it to *support* a process designed to arrive at a decision? Or ...

B) Was it to *support* a decision already made?

In the former, this tool may serve as a useful, supplemental source to help guide sound decision-making. Though imperfect, it didn't seem improper. Many businesses and industries use data to assist in strategic planning and decision quality.

Examining and comparing achievement to goals, metric-specific improvements/declines over time, and individual, unit, and group performance is hard to do without a set of tools and methods by which these tools should be used.

In the latter, it appeared a method by which the ends were justified by the means.

With certainty, I didn't know which applied here. I wondered, however, how this TPA figured out *all* that they purported, in twenty questions, without ever seeing, touching, or talking to a patient?

Fascinating. And to some degree—maybe only for me—frightening.

BCBS's "partner" introduction and it's predictive outcome report produced one *real* thing that bears additional commentary, as it directly relates to a topic highlighted in a previous chapter.

With its projected discharge date—answering the question, *When can I go home?*—there was a potentially massive problem with creating, and subsequently managing, patient and family expectations:

What if the date when the patient can go home—was wrong?

Would it be wrong because of something …

- The patient did/didn't do?
- The family did/didn't do?
- The physician, nurse, or therapist did/didn't do?
- The predictive decision-support tool didn't do?

Probably not …

It would be wrong because of something the nursing home did/didn't do.

Regardless of duration, a patient experiences plenty between these three milestones:

- Their last day hospitalized, before their nursing home admission
- Their nursing home admission day
- Their last day in the nursing home before being discharged

These experiences can be very un-*predict*-able.

Yet once the TPA projects the patient's discharge date, it's seared into their (and their family's) consciousness. Might as well be a guarantee.

Indisputable, incontrovertible, unassailable.

The very best work in concurrent review or continuing authorizations will not unmanage that expectation. Someone will be on the hook if the projected discharge date—established on, before, or near to Day One of a patient's nursing home stay—isn't successfully met.

These were my thoughts, on a single issue, related to the TPA's use of answers to "twenty questions."

Hey ... isn't there a *game* with this same name?

ꕥ

Before leaving this topic, I'll add additional context for consideration. Instead of examining it through the nursing home's lens, we'll view it as a patient or family member.

In the process, we'll find additional hidden truths which impede a patient's chance to win. Imagine, for a moment, the challenges and anxieties accompanying this experience:

You're a nursing home patient, admitted after a fall at home and a two-day hospital stay.

In a seventy-two-hour span, you were injured, went from your home to a hospital, then to a nursing home. You didn't plan this. Don't know how it happened. You're scared.

At or near the time of admission, you learn from the nursing home that your Medicare Advantage plan has predicted your length of stay to be fourteen days, after which they'll stop payment to the nursing home, since you'll be ready to go home.

When you're ready to go home, their plan is for you to receive home health for continued care. Someone will visit to provide treatment, consistent with your specific skilled care needs as assessed, predicted, and ultimately determined by the health plan.

The health plan has *projected* the amount of time and home health services you'll need after you're discharged to home. When this projection is met, the health plan will discontinue payment for home health services. This is because they're projecting that you will be good to go.

It's now *Day Eleven* in your nursing home stay. You're sore from participating in therapy for several hours each day and still trying to figure out what exactly happened to you. You hate the food, have had two total strangers as roommates, and haven't had a decent night's sleep since the day before you fell at home.

In seventy-two hours, you're going home. You're still scared, lacking confidence, and aren't ready to go. Even with visits from the kindest and most caring home health workers, you'll still be *alone* for most of every day, fearing for your own safety.

Now ... you're screwed. The health plan is on track to discontinue payment to the nursing home. The nursing home isn't going to challenge the health plan, as this places their relationship with the plan at risk. You're not ready to go home, and your world is moving very quickly.

Your options are:

- **Appeal the decision made by the health plan.** If you do, the wait might be long. Health plans likely won't treat this as an emergency, even though it is to you.
- **Pay for your continued nursing home stay.** Now, you have to figure out how. Cash? Credit card? Apply for Medicaid? Understandably, the nursing home will want to have security around continued payment.

One can argue—and I have many times—that arrangements for secondary (or contingent) payment sources should have been made at the time, or shortly after, a patient's admission. But ... this isn't easy, and takes time to do correctly.

Family members are scared and have their hands full with the similar challenges. They're spectators in a game whose rules are unfamiliar. Yet, the clock continues to run, and the reliance on the *projections* made by the health plan have become bedrock.

In their minds, if the health plan *said* that the patient can *go home* in two weeks, there shouldn't have been any reason to worry about payment on *Day Fifteen*. Right?

I mean, the health plan said so!

Now what? The date when the patient *should* go home—is wrong. The patient and family feel that they have been lied to. Now, they begin desperately searching for the truth ... and someone to blame.

Myth #5—"Patient-Centric" Means Patients Benefit

Having explored structural and functional hidden truths, let's pivot to the administrative and bureaucratic, where deficits in industrial experience among decision-makers make the truth sometimes hard to find—resulting in people being hurt badly.

When gubernatorial administrations are challenged in their budgeting, unpopular things happen—like increased fees and increased taxes. These reelection killers, even among the term-limited, follow politicians seeking higher office and can serve as their party's legacy in future electoral challenges.

Politicians know this history and do everything to avoid it. It's a mistaken perception that elected officials and their policymakers aren't smart. They are. Very.

So instead of embracing programs likely to tarnish their legacies, or their party's, state leaders will build and drive programs that appear to be "for the people" and end up not really being so.

Here's an example befitting this definition.

Minnesota's Medicaid program has a benefit for nursing home patients called *desired therapeutic leave*, providing patients the ability to take a "home visit, vacation, or other therapeutic leave" from a nursing home, and the requirements which homes must follow in program administration.[40]

Program highlights include:

- Patient overnight absences "of more than twenty-three hours and any subsequent consecutive calendar days."
- Homes can bill for these days if their occupancy during the month is "equal to or greater than 96 percent."
- If occupancy is less than 96 percent, *and* the patient chooses not to pay for their leave days, the nursing home

may opt to involuntarily discharge the patient, subject to a thirty-day advance notice of discharge.

- If the home "elects not to discharge ... and waives the leave day payment, this policy needs to be applied to all ... in similar circumstances, regardless of payment source."
- Under certain circumstances, if patients are discharged from the home, they have the right to be readmitted to the first available, same-sex, semiprivate bed.

Nursing homes support the notion of patients leaving for overnights and—if desired—for consecutive days (and nights). Patients should be able to attend a grandchild's high school or college graduation, celebrate a wedding or anniversary, or create memories that add quality to their life.

Prohibiting homes from billing Medicaid for a held bed—unless they're nearly full—isn't an issue either. This has been an industrial standard for years, and it's inarguable that a state pay to reserve a bed in a home that is insufficiently occupied.

Things begin to unravel, however, regarding involuntarily discharging patients with a thirty-day notice regardless of payor source. Program architects know these facts:

- Medicaid patients *can't* afford to pay the nursing home for their bed to be held while on therapeutic leave.
- Private paying patients *aren't* going to pay for a bed to be held, and know that.
- Nursing homes *won't* involuntarily discharge patients and risk the pain and punishment—from assorted agencies—associated with an equal (or unequal) application of the payment waiver provision.

Congratulations are in order for this *Dogs on Velvet*-like creation by budget analysts and agency representatives. On a macro level, it provided nursing home patients a vacation from living in a home, protected their rights and bank accounts, and saved their state a tremendous amount of money.

How much? Most likely, it's millions annually.

A recent report from the Minnesota Department of Human Services indicated the average daily Medicaid rate for a Minnesota nursing home patient is $373.[41] Reducing by 25 percent—for wiggle room—the daily revenue hit for one therapeutic leave day is $280.

To fortify this projection, a nursing home patient receives thirty-six therapeutic leave days annually in Minnesota:

Yes, 3-6. Let's do the math on this, calculating the revenue lost by the nursing home and saved by the state:

# OF PATIENTS USING LEAVE DAYS	LOST REVENUE/ DAY*	LOST REVENUE W/36 DAYS USED
1	$280	$10,080
10	$2,800	$100,800
100	$28,000	$1,008,000

**Using an artificially deflated $280/day average Medicaid rate*

Patients that are able, and fluent with program parameters, use their therapeutic leave days, taking more than one or two at a time.

Truth is, patients take them in bunches, many times going solo, contrary to the imagery of accompanying family members for a reunion, wedding, graduation, or barbecue. This is based on experiences with homes in Minnesota and extensive conversations with very talented people paid to care for and protect these patients.

People who live in or frequently visit Minnesota also know this: Their weather *sucks*. Unless, of course, you love to snowmobile, hunt, ice fish, watch outdoor hockey games, or own a snowplowing business. It can snow in May, and probably will snow in September. The mosquitos up there could probably eat pork chops.

Nursing home patients, who don't keep Wolverine boots and Canada Goose jackets in their closets, know this too. They take their therapeutic leave days during nice weather, like June through August.

I've heard stories of patients taking therapeutic leaves for two-to-three uninterrupted weeks. Returning to their nursing home after their time away ... they're often really f*cked up.

Like people who go on a cruise and gain fifteen pounds, or go to Vegas and come back broke (or broken), these nursing home patients will go unmonitored. Medically, nutritionally, and psychosocially. Prior progress or routines established via their plans of care ... evaporate. *Poof!*

Medication management isn't the nursing home's responsibility while the patient is on leave. Think for a moment what happens to a younger, ambulatory, willful nursing home patient who misses a day (or two ... or ten) of their prescribed antipsychotics. Now, who are you most scared for—the patient, or those who the patient might encounter while on therapeutic leave?

This is what happens when no one's paid to care.

In one company, we encouraged our homes to stay connected with patients taking multiday or multiweek therapeutic leaves. Offering free breakfasts, lunches, and dinners were opportunities to "check in" and have medications administered ... before going back out to play.

Successful? Not even close. Once out on leave, even nursing home patients don't want to be in a nursing home.

When the weather sucks—again—patients will return to their respective homes. Some earlier than anticipated and others not. Once back in the building, it's easy to imagine the behavioral challenges from patients now having had their *freedom* taken away. There are times when it takes only a single patient to disturb or destroy the living environment for every other patient within a nursing home.

This one policy item, alone—and the truths not found in the state's health department guidance—makes working and living in a Minnesota nursing home hard. And for patient care continuity, it can be a losing proposition where people get hurt—and badly.

Myth #6—A Medicaid Patient Is a Medicaid Patient Is a Medicaid Patient ...

Collisions—of bureaucratically-driven policies and nursing home decision-makers—create environments fraught with risk, where truths aren't known until it's far too late.

On its face, Medicaid recipients—based solely on asset and income eligibility criteria—possess financial similarities. Additionally, limited marketplace leverage and reliance on this program for their *existence* are common denominators.

This is where their common ground ends.

No two Medicaid patients are alike. In fact, their differences can be considerable. Differences which create complexity and risks, leading to danger—and harm.

Differences, between older and much, much younger Medicaid patients, involving people who absolutely don't want to live in a nursing home yet have fallen through every crack imaginable before finding it their residence of last resort.

Their histories include work, sex, and choices—good, bad, or in-between. Friendships made and extinguished. Children. Mourning. Rejection—from partners, spouses, and parents. Money and freedoms lost.

Bringing their unchecked baggage to the nursing home, it often includes having lost their thirties, forties, or fifties—with dimmed prospects ahead.

Acronyms accompany younger patients and their baggage, including:

- CVA — Cerebrovascular accident or stroke
- MVA — Motor vehicle accident
- BKA — Below-the-knee amputation
- GSW — Gunshot wound

Their stories and conditions can be the result of being in the wrong place at the wrong time, mismanagement of underlying medical conditions (e.g., diabetes), acute or chronic narcotics use, or incredibly bad luck.

Men and women, from sixteen to sixty.

Early on, each rapidly learns they're living in a place incompatible with meeting their nonmedical needs. Residents' rights, while favorable to patients, can *never* compete with the freedoms enjoyed by people outside an institutional setting. Rules regarding visiting hours, overnight guests, smoking, and alcohol are examples where nursing home policies, bureaucratically-driven regulations, and personal preferences collide.

Like any other, when needs go unmet—patients get angry. When they've checked in—angry or regretful, due to loss, abandonment, fear, loneliness, or self-loathing—they can become angrier.

And a threat to other patients.

I've read incident reports of patient-to-patient encounters where people have been severely injured. I've viewed recorded incidents—as an executive and expert—where the violence is on par with anything you'd see on a streaming channel.

Concussions, lacerations, broken bones, sexual assault. Using their hands, fists, feet, sharp and blunt objects.

These incidents don't involve action heroes or stunt doubles, but everyday people. Many times the victim doesn't see what's coming.

Like what is shared in news or online—on streets, parking lots, and playgrounds, and in school classrooms and hallways—these events are stunning, upsetting, and unnecessary. Yet they happen.

My mom was a victim of patient-to-patient violence. I vividly remember receiving the phone call on the night it occurred. Learning that Mom had been punched in her face by a male patient, I had two questions for the evening supervisor on the other end:

"Can you please send me a picture of Mom?"

"What does the other guy look like?"

Within minutes and before the call's conclusion, I received a picture of my mother, smiling, with a fresh welt on her cheek and the remnants of a bloodied nose. Seeing this was infuriating, heartbreaking, somewhat understandable, and many, many years later—somewhat amusing.

And the other guy? While HIPAA regulations prohibited me from getting a look at his mug shot, the supervisor shared that he got a whole lot more than what he'd bargained for when he tried to go fifteen rounds with Mom. She drew blood and got in more shots than received. Before Mom was finished with him, he was in full retreat.

That old man never screwed with Ann Davis again. *Nor did anyone else.*

My mom's case differs from the gaps between older and younger patients. Her attacker was an older gentleman, and occurred in a memory care facility where no real generational gaps existed. In a nursing home, however, the environment is remarkably different, age gaps are readily apparent, and nursing home decision-makers contribute heavily to risks and their intensity.

You see, when homes are experiencing challenges to occupancy and profitability, they'll communicate to the market (e.g., hospitals and referral sources) that they're committed to *"taking anything,"* commoditizing by condition rather than personalizing patients. With each passing day that a nursing home fails to meet or exceed their *targets,* or occupancy and earnings goals, sales and operations incentives and bonuses diminish.

Referral sources will take them at their word, working to transfer patients that these homes—in retrospect—wished they'd never considered.

In fairness, my nursing home experiences—since the 1980s—included providing care to the old and the not-so-old. These experiences, however, also included establishing limits on the number and condition of younger patients, for reasons shared earlier.

While touring homes across the nation, I'd intentionally count the number of patients under fifty. At the tour's conclusion, I'd share my count of younger patients and ask the home's leadership—"What are you doing for these people?"

Smoking and alcohol use among all nursing home patients are daily challenges regardless of a patient's age. Even in smoke- and alcohol-free homes, patients can creatively find solutions to prohibition.

Just like we might have when we were kids.

With younger patients, these and other dimensions make individual and population management very hard for a nursing home.

Like commingling students by grade in primary and secondary education, there are always situations where groups or grades of students are stronger and more powerful than others. This is equally true in nursing homes that commingle younger and stronger patients among the older and infirm. Add a dose of anger and frustration, plus a steady diet of the words *NO* or *STOP*, and the environment is ripe for scary experiences involving patients who can deliver punishment and those unable to defend against this threat.

Contrary to beliefs of some, a person's sexual desires are not always vacated due to disability or infirmity. Pick an age and try to remember the desires that captivated you. Younger nursing home patients experience these same feelings. Some will enjoy the company of visitors, paid or unpaid. Others will seek companionship from others affiliated with the nursing home—among consenting patients or workers, present or former. In extremely unfortunate situations, they'll inflict harm on other patients, out of frustration, the absence of treatment, or being placed in an environment for which they are totally unsuited.

When this happens, the truth is—there are no winners. Just losers.

ᔕ

Unfortunately, the risks associated with younger patients don't end here. Because of illness, unchecked baggage, policy, and competing social priorities, younger patients can be a threat to themselves.

The intersection of patients' rights and the electronic age has made monitoring and controlling the trafficking of narcotics among younger nursing home patients a daily management nightmare. Patients have their own phones, make and receive calls, text, and conduct private business transactions.

"Stop and Frisk" is a no-go in a nursing home. If a patient can procure and secure it, nursing home leadership can find their hands tied, forced to manage the aftermath—or hope that a patient inadvertently leaves their "stash" in their clothes sent to the laundry, or stuffed inside their wheelchair when it's scheduled for cleaning.

When these lucky bounces don't occur, results can be catastrophic. Here's one story where sex, drugs, and money resulted in a very sad day for one nursing home and a young patient under their care.

This downtown nursing home was located on a busy thoroughfare. With zero-setback from the street, it could be entered from the city's sidewalk—something one might not always think of when envisioning a typical nursing home.

Traffic past the nursing home was constant during daylight and evening hours. A bus stop was nearby, yet the street directly in front of the home was dedicated to metered parking. Pedestrians routinely walked past the building, communicating with patients whose daily routine included hanging out near the home's entrance.

Licensed as a nursing home, this wasn't a typical setting. It specialized in providing care to younger patients, who were active in every way imaginable. Each patient had care needs that couldn't be satisfied with community-based resources. Many had treatment histories where this had been attempted—and failed.

This market had no state hospital system, or an infrastructure designed specifically to treat patients whose needs required mental health services. The nursing home bridged this service gap through a combination of on-site Qualified Intellectual Disability Professionals (QIDP), attending physicians, consulting psychiatrists, and psychiatric social workers.

I'm sharing this story to illustrate that even in homes with competent, capable, and experienced leadership and programming designed to provide the best care possible for younger patients, incredibly bad things happen.

It involved a woman in her mid-forties, a patient of this nursing home for over a year. Her life's history included alcohol and drug abuse, many relationships ending in distress, and multiple hospitalizations due to self-abuse or injuries sustained at the hands of others.

Her nursing home stay had been uneventful. She exercised her freedom to leave the home as desired, always returning and never exhibiting an elopement risk. She participated in her treatment plan, took medications as prescribed, and met her physicians and therapists as scheduled.

As a Medicaid patient, she received a monthly stipend, which was deposited into her Personal Needs Account.

Unbeknownst to many, this woman had resumed her former lifestyle; she would exit the home and enter parked cars for the purpose of providing sex in return for cash.

When this behavior became suspected, and confirmed, it placed the nursing home in a difficult position. Since this activity took place outside the nursing home, the home's leadership was required to respect the rights afforded this person. Any surveillance or intervention by the nursing home on this city's street was an invasion of the patient's privacy and could place a nursing home worker at risk of bodily harm.

Local police had limited interest, as the city had numerous competing priorities for public safety, which didn't include oversight of something that *might happen, at an undetermined time*, involving a nursing home patient.

It would be improper to speculate in a number of areas involving this sad story, and we'll stick to facts which include that the frequency of this behavior was dependent on weather, the patient's daily condition, and pedestrian traffic. When it was very hot or cold, she wasn't feeling well, or the streets were busy with foot traffic, this patient spent more time inside the home than out.

Nevertheless, high-risk behavior is newsworthy in communities, and this was no exception. Over time, illicit drugs became an alternative currency for services, and this patient was being paid in a combination of cash and heroin.

One day, the nursing home learned about this latter payment form only after it was too late.

Returning to the home after spending time on the street, this patient boarded an elevator, rode it to the floor where her room was located, and injected herself with enough heroin to induce death.

Found by a worker in one of the home's community bathrooms, the needle used was beside her. Attempts to revive were unsuccessful.

A true and sad story, this is.

Myth #7—The Fine Print Doesn't Matter

It would have been easy to end this chapter here, highlighting hidden truths impacting nursing home patients and hospitals, taxpayer-funded programs, insurance companies, lawmakers, and bureaucrats. This information might have been surprising and hard to handle.

But this chapter intends to inform. And to help readers be better decision-makers and *advocates* for themselves and loved ones.

Over the next few pages, we'll explore one final set of hidden truths, hoping they provoke thought, preparing *you* to be a more well-informed advocate.

Search for "organizations that advocate for senior citizens" and you'll find nonprofit agencies like the National Council on Aging, Justice in Aging, the American Society on Aging, and others whose mission is devoted to protecting or improving the lives of those who've been around awhile.

These are welcomed groups. If you've ever said, or had directed to you, the comment (or retort), "OK, Boomer," or have been referred to as "old," this is code enough to figure out that organizations looking out for us geezers are OK.

During this same search were blogger-generated articles and other items like these:

- "15 Organizations Working to Advocate for Seniors"[42]
- "Check Out These Organizations That Help Senior Citizens"[43]

The number one draft choice among advocacy groups cited by these authors was AARP, formerly known as the American Association of Retired Persons. The group most often presumed to *have the backs of seniors*—on Capitol Hill in Washington, DC, and in each of the fifty states and territories. Their message to members and the public:

"We're in your community—advocating for you on important issues and providing a range of opportunities to learn, connect, and have fun."[44]

What they are doing—on behalf of seniors—matters. Boomers and older Americans feel the effects of their work—*now*. Younger generations, especially those approaching their fifties, will soon follow.

If you've visited a medical practice in the past—say, thirty years—you know AARP. Their magazines are simply gorgeous. Celebrities who look better now than they did in their twenties grace their covers. Bold colors are found throughout these publications, and the seniors displayed inside look almost as good as the superstars on the cover.

Yes. That magazine. If you're in your forties, or older, you know them from the monthly or quarterly mailer that you look at once and toss with fliers from retailers and insurance agents that you don't know, and never will.

AARP has an estimated *thirty-eight million* members.[45] That's a lot of geezers.

Though I've been over fifty for a while, and still receiving their mailers, I've never been an AARP member. No, the $16 annual membership rate isn't the deal-breaker. Their content, platform, and practices are.

Let me explain. Years ago, when my wife was a member and receiving their monthly magazine, I'd flip through them. One day, I stopped.

Why? It wasn't because of the recipes, or travel and lifestyle stuff. It was because of the advocacy—at least by the way it was being presented.

Sorting through messaging buried in their printed materials, I concluded:

AARP was *in the tank* with insurance companies.

Broadway Joe, Captain Kirk, and King of *Dy-No-Mite!* … move over. This group was a much bigger machine than what these guys could ever be on their ninety-second, late-night, promos.

Studying articles written about Medicare and Medicare Advantage, each seemingly possessed a tone leaning heavily toward Medicare Advantage. In some cases, relative comparisons of strengths versus weaknesses and evaluations of plans were partially—or fully—excluded.

Granted, I recognize my own biases. One massive difference, however, is that *I'm not being paid to influence*—overtly or by tilt—one path over another. It can be argued, however, that *AARP*—self-described as "a wise friend and fierce defender, focusing on the priorities of older Americans"[46] …

Is.

ဢ

Yeah, my opinion-based shade is being thrown at this advocacy group, whose magazine sports face-men and women whose Q-ratings are off the charts within their readers' age groups.

For-profit companies could learn a lot from AARP's marketing and market research.

So why is it that I'm throwing the high, hard one at this group? Is it because I don't like their magazine?

Nope.

No, this opinion stems largely from the belief that AARP has crossed the line on this equation:

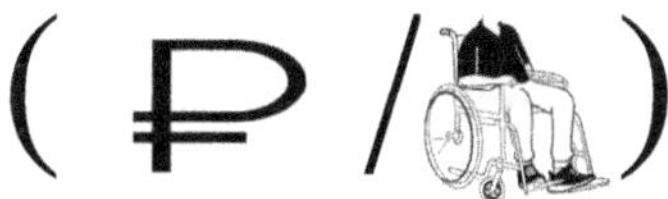

Source: Dave Devereaux

This is my illustration of *Profits over People*. Yes, this math is not limited to nursing homes. Here's why …

On www.aarpmedicareplans.com, you'll find this sentence near the page's bottom:

"UnitedHealthcare Insurance Company pays royalty fees to AARP for the use of its intellectual property. These fees are used for the general purposes of AARP."[47]

Pretty benign, yes? *Royalty fee* ... Yeah, *maybe*.

Search for "AARP Medicare Supplement" and you'll find a cobranded promotion between AARP and UnitedHealthcare. Accompanied by this fine print:

"AARP endorses the AARP Medicare Supplement Insurance Plans. Insurers of the Plan pay royalty fees to AARP for the use of its intellectual property. These fees are used for the general purposes of AARP. AARP and its affiliates are not insurers. AARP does not employ or endorse agents, brokers, or producers."[48]

Finally, while searching for AARP Medicare Rx Plans, you'll find "AARP Medicare® Rx Plans from UnitedHealthcare®." And to learn more about the plan, "You'll leave AARP and go to the website of a trusted third-party. The third-party's terms, conditions, and policies apply."[49]

So … what does this royalty fee and trusted third-party relationship amount to?

An April 24, 2024, special report prepared by Chris Jacobs, "How AARP's Profits Harm Patients—And Violate Its Principles" examines

AARP's business practices and the challenges resulting from their relationship with UnitedHealth Group (UHG), among others.

In it, Jacobs reports:

- For decades, AARP's prime source of revenue has come through its relationship with UnitedHealth.
- Since 2007, AARP has received an estimated $9 billion, tax-free, from UnitedHealth.
- Since 2009, AARP's net profits totaled nearly $2.1 billion, notching gains in all but one of those fourteen years.[50]

Maybe this royalty fee isn't so benign after all.

The fine print shared from AARP's website (which no one reads, except people doing research) indicates that these royalty fees are used "for the general purposes of AARP," which means:

We can do whatever we want with them.

Additionally, Jacobs highlights AARP's advocacy for legislative efforts that have completely hosed old people and torpedoed Medicare, including the Inflation Reduction Act and Obamacare.

For people clinging to the notion that non-for-profits struggle financially because doing good exhausts donation and foundation grant funding, these next points may be particularly salient.

AARP's annual financial highlights, reported by Jacobs, per their 2022 IRS Form 990, indicated:[51]

TOTAL REVENUES	**$1.8 BILLION**
Membership Dues Revenue	$291 million (16.1% of total)
Royalty Fees (use of logo, brand, IP)	$1.1 billion
Net Income	$91.3 million

Figures for recent years are calculated approximations, because "beginning in 2018, AARP's consolidated financial statements *failed to disclose* the exact percentage of its marketing revenue from UnitedHealth."[52] (emphasis added).

Meaning, information that wasn't previously hidden, now is. Not even in fine print.

Prior to this darkness, AARP's financials could be examined with precision. Additionally, citing Jacobs:

- 2007 revenues from UnitedHealth represented *57 percent* of AARPs marketing income, or *$283 million*.
- By 2017, revenues from UnitedHealth comprised *69 percent* of AARP's marketing revenue and had risen to *$627.2 million*—more than double the amount from just a decade previously."[53]

AARP's (via UnitedHealth) financial improvement tracks nicely with the nation's Medicare Advantage growth (in millions) as indicated in the graph, *"Annual Medicare Advantage Enrollment."* While this illustration is similar to that shared earlier, it's based on number—rather than percentage—of plan participants.[54]

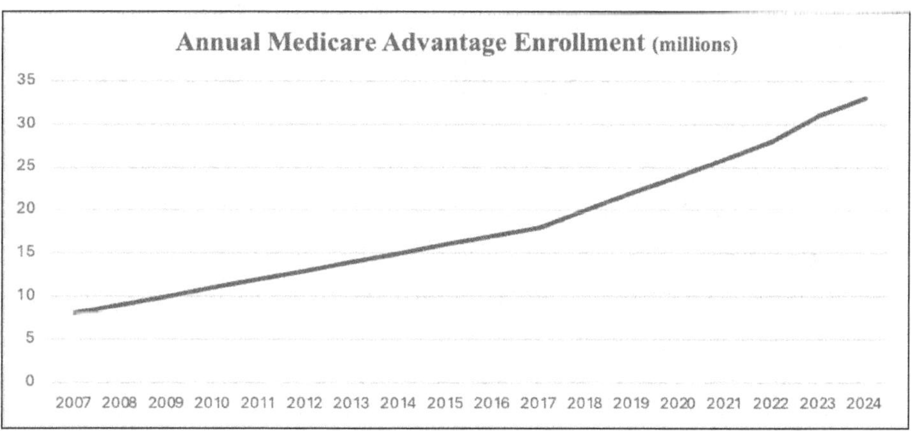

So … money AARP might be receiving through marketing deals with Avis, Budget, Best Western, Choice Hotels, or Bonefish Grill is likely not dominating their business attention. Most likely, their insurance marketing relationship, royalty fee, and trusted third-party relationship with UnitedHealth …

Is.

Wrapping up here, it's worth wondering … Is all this wrong? There are all kinds of marketing companies that get a taste of what they sell to their membership from their trusted third parties or authorized dealers.

For me, questions revolve around *advocacy*. Business arrangements with an insurance heavyweight champion. Publishing material that members may unknowingly rely upon involving complex and personal topics—like healthcare and insurance. A dearth of disclosure around sources and uses of cash.

It's easy to wonder if, what type, or how many conflicts of interest this first-round draft choice among senior advocates is perceived to be in—or at least coming very close to.

Regardless, the optics aren't pretty.

Too much to consider? Maybe. I'll share this. It's hard for me to know exactly what the truth might be. Is the *advocate of advocates* working on behalf of its senior members—or at their expense? Said differently, do they *have the backs of seniors*?

I think the fine print tells this story. You can decide—are they open secrets, or hidden truths?

WHAT YOU CAN DO

Ask Questions About:

- Money. It's nothing to be afraid of. Ask *everyone*:
    - What will it cost?
    - Are discounts available?
    - When is payment required—before, at the time of, or following service?

    - Whose money gets used first—and last?
    - How are benefits (insurance) coordinated in payment?
    - What happens if the money runs out?

- Coverage, eligibility, and what happens after neither continue to apply?
- ... *and then what?* Keep asking this question until you have everything answered.
- Treatment approaches based on payor source. Do tiers influence behaviors?
- Applying the standard for care equally, regardless of tier or payor.

Look for:

- Fine print. If they wrote it, it's worth reading. Especially really fine print.
- Affiliated partnerships and cobranding. Who gets what, from whom, and why?

Listen to What People Say:

- Clichés or Specifics? Which do speakers use when discussing important things?
- Are people communicating only what they *think* you want to hear?

IV

LIFE(STYLE)-SUSTAINING MACHINERY

Relative to other industries, nursing homes are low-tech businesses. Most work, transactionally rooted, is performed by people. Bathing and clothing patients. Preparing meals. Repairing and maintaining equipment.

Yet homes rely on machinery to fully complete, or assist, in daily tasks. Monitoring vital signs and changes in condition. Assisting in recovery and rehabilitation. Sharing informatics among multiple departments. Preparing billing and financial statements.

Other machines directly provide oxygen, liquid nutrition, or medication to patients. Without it, caring for people would be harder. In some cases, impossible. In these latter examples, machines are bridges to sustaining life.

The Machinery

Today's nursing home business also relies on other machinery.

On its surface, it involves separate, distinct relationships between one tenant and one landlord, each owned by common parties.

Only on paper.

The rest, while entirely legal when structured properly, is frequently BS.

In nursing home ownership structures, an operating company (OpCo) carries the nursing home's *operating* license. Their success is dependent on the performance of the nursing home's daily operations and reliant on the skills, talent, creativity, and approach of the people working for the home, or OpCo.

While the OpCo is licensed to run the nursing home, it owns very little. Under oath, owners frequently purport that an OpCo is responsible for *everything* at a nursing home yet owns *nothing* associated with it.

Conversely, a real estate or property company (PropCo) carries the mortgage on the nursing home and manages everything related to the nursing home as a tangible, physical asset—land, bricks and mortar, and many things inside it. In other words, the *property* in its entirety. These same owners will argue that a PropCo owns *everything* about a nursing home yet does *nothing* beyond what's required of a real estate owner.

This machine intentionally makes people cross-eyed. It's designed to prevent concrete answers about *who's accountable for what* within a nursing home.

OpCos, sometimes without *any* employees, will farm out responsibility for daily decision-making to a management company (ManCo). ManCos—frequently owned by the same parties as OpCos and PropCos—employ people who work with, *not for*, the nursing home, like subject-matter experts, consultants, and supervisors of nursing home administrators.

By fee agreement with the OpCo, ManCos provide support or back-of-the house services found in all business types (e.g., billing, legal, insurance), providing scale and economy beyond what a nursing home can achieve on its own.

This briefly illustrates OpCo behavior with its PropCo and ManCo:

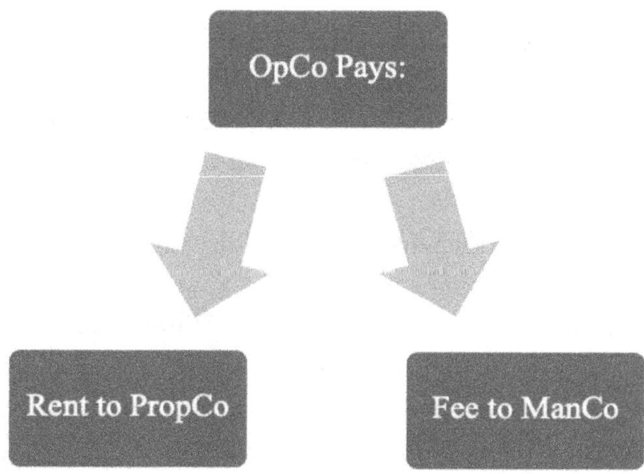

This summarizes the machinery parts, in grid-format:

OPERATING COMPANY (OPCO)	MANAGEMENT COMPANY (MANCO)	PROPERTY COMPANY (PROPCO)
Holds the nursing home's license	Subcontracted by the OpCo	Separate from the OpCo and the ManCo
Manages the nursing home	Paid management fee by the OpCo	Carries the nursing home's mortgage
Pays rent to the PropCo and fee to the ManCo	Provides services to the nursing home	Leases home to the OpCo
Owns very little	Owns virtually nothing	Owns the nursing home

Yes, this ManCo wrinkle is also intentional, further obscuring responsibilities by business entity. Even with common ownership—across OpCo, PropCo, and ManCo—it's difficult to identify *who's accountable for what* within a nursing home.

And that's how nursing home owners like it.

A Closer Look Inside

OK, what's this all mean and why should you care? It's like learning who was behind the curtain in *The Wizard of Oz*.

Among nursing home companies providing public access to names, faces, and titles of owners and executives via websites, it's easy to identify those whose responsibilities rest with an OpCo, a PropCo, or a ManCo.

Owners, founders, principals, managing directors, CEOs, CFOs, CAOs, and others will have headshots on company websites highlighting dual responsibilities and titles. Some companies attempt to fake out consumers, displaying titles and biographies on their separate PropCo, financial management, and investment company or group (InvestCo) pages, while going dark on anything related to their OpCos.

However, press releases, published articles and interviews, and observed behaviors, make the BS smoke screen less overwhelming ... *ish.*

Here's another grid that should help:

Employment—by Entity

OPCO	MANCO	PROPCO
Nursing home administrator	Field operations middle/sr. mgmt.	Very, very few
Director of nursing	Nursing consultants	
Nursing home department leaders	Subject-matter experts	
Nursing home workers	Other support for home(s)	

If you're struggling to follow how these entities—and people—fit together, I'll share my work experience. As a nursing home administrator, I was employed and paid by an OpCo. In larger roles associated with managing multiple homes, a division, or a nursing home company, I was employed by a ManCo.

And after all these years, I've still yet to meet someone employed and paid by a PropCo.

Financial Engineering

In these arrangements, owners, founders, and other financial *engineers* determined what and how much an OpCo was billed for the costs of running their businesses, including rent, insurance, and management fees.

Companies might assign nursing homes their expenses based on internally determined formulas, rather than invoices and receipts of home-specific purchases. In others, financial engineers would forgo assigning expenses to homes, obscuring financial performance shared with interested parties.

This behavior is frequently due to the maniacal pursuit of government-backed financing, provided by the US Department of Housing and Urban Development (HUD). With HUD financing, owners and investors are repaid their initial investments, providing fuel for future deals.

More importantly, HUD financing is nonrecourse[55]—simultaneously replacing initial owner and investor funding, and terminating any personal guarantee of financial solvency.

When nursing home owners default on nonrecourse HUD financing due to management misadventures, market shifts, poor strategic planning and execution caused by deficient patient care quality, litigation, or financial penalties connected with survey outcomes, their responsibility—under this arrangement—is simply to return the keys to the building.

Contrary to recourse loans, where borrowers are personally responsible for remaining loan balances not satisfied by collateral, owners and investors applying for nonrecourse HUD financing never have to make up the outstanding loan balance when things go *tilt*.

Quite a deal … if you can get it.

This absence of recourse gives financial engineers tremendous latitude in their decision-making. Risks become structurally unbalanced. When homes are driven to financial ruin, patients, workers, and the community suffer. Owners don't.

And that's how nursing home owners like it.

Today, in an industry with minimal public reporting requirements, approaches taken by OpCos and PropCos can defy logic.

Behaviors toward achieving profitability are inverted. I've worked for some where OpCo profitability through performance was a secondary (or tertiary) short- and long-term concern.

Strategically, they sought to enjoy the benefits produced by their *related-party ancillary businesses*, rather than their core businesses—the nursing homes' operations.

In these cases, related-party businesses, paid directly by OpCos for their services, received little governmental oversight, or internal governance. Nevertheless, they provided consistently healthy distributions to owners and investors.

Without competitive bidding or market consideration, prices nursing homes paid to related parties were established by financial engineers. Quality and competence required only small hurdles be cleared by its leadership, whether it be the ability to fog a mirror with exhaled breath, or a direct linkage to owners.

The goal of this arrangement?

Weaken the OpCo, and sustain the PropCo. For common owners of both, enjoy the tax advantage associated with the losses of the former to offset any gains—current or future—associated with the latter.

Complicated? Yeah, maybe. Very good tax accountants sort this stuff out with ease.

And when these business arrangements are fully exploited, with OpCo financial statements reflecting losses or poor performance, they seek lifelines to maintain their *machinery*. Lifelines, sought by lobbyists and trade association representatives, created by lawmakers, and paid for by taxpayers.

Financial Dialysis

This chapter's opening described machines—like oxygen concentrators and intravenous pumps—as bridges to sustaining patients' lives. While their features may be technologically complex, their purpose is incredibly simple.

Though organizationally and structurally complex, *the financial machinery of nursing homes* has an equally simple purpose. Rather than providing patients with life-sustaining services, its purpose is to provide a *lifestyle-sustaining* service to its owners and investors.

Fueling their engines—are nursing home patients. A constant flow of them. Without patients, this *machinery* breaks.

We'll focus on what this machinery does in providing *lifestyle-sustaining* services to many nursing home owners and investors.

I call it *financial dialysis.*

At the risk of offending your sensibilities, there are nursing home owners and executives for whom *dialyzing dollars through the body of each patient* are core strategies.

Offended? Consider this batting practice.

To those who benefit most, nursing homes are the oxygen supply to their coveted related-party businesses.

Patients. People. Parents and grandparents. Friends and relatives. Bodies and benefits.

∽

Nursing homes, through their sales forces, beg endlessly for patients. They beg because it's an outgrowth of their real or perceived status as being perpetually—and industrially—impoverished.

Concretely defining the word *poor* is elusive. It's a relative term. Compared to what? Compared to whom? And for how long? Answers lie *only* between the ears and eyes of the individual.

My observations, across decades in this business, are that individuals define themselves as poor relative to others. When this occurs, erasing any taint of having less—comparatively speaking—becomes a priority.

Even when the absolute value of their incomes and net worth places them firmly in the category of the top 1 percent or truly rich people, internal relative value scales make it impossible to see themselves as anything approaching this distinction.

As a result, *maximize* becomes the word to remember—and repeat to others. I'll share that after twenty-five years of pain and punishment, in courts and with state and federal regulators, industry power brokers and their surrogates—who have been taught and know better—still choose *maximize* over the preferred and advised substitute, *optimize.*

This isn't a word game. Behaviors in achieving the former differ when compared to the latter.

Consider this, briefly. In baseball, pitchers are routinely evaluated on the speed (miles per hour) of their fastball. The construct is, the faster the ball is thrown (or moves), the more attractive—or profitable—the pitcher or prospect might be to a team.

At least until the pursuit of *maximizing* speed results in the pitcher losing control of where the ball goes—in which case batters gain the advantage. Increasing speed eventually has diminishing returns, or results in injury, each of which can be a liability.

OK, back to the nursing home business, the machine, and financial dialysis ...

When patients are put through financial dialysis, *maximization* attempts to convert the flesh, blood, bone, muscle, time, energy, and spirit of every patient into as many dollars for as many related-party businesses as possible.

This is a sample illustration of financial dialysis machinery, with nursing home patients as input for related-party ancillary businesses:

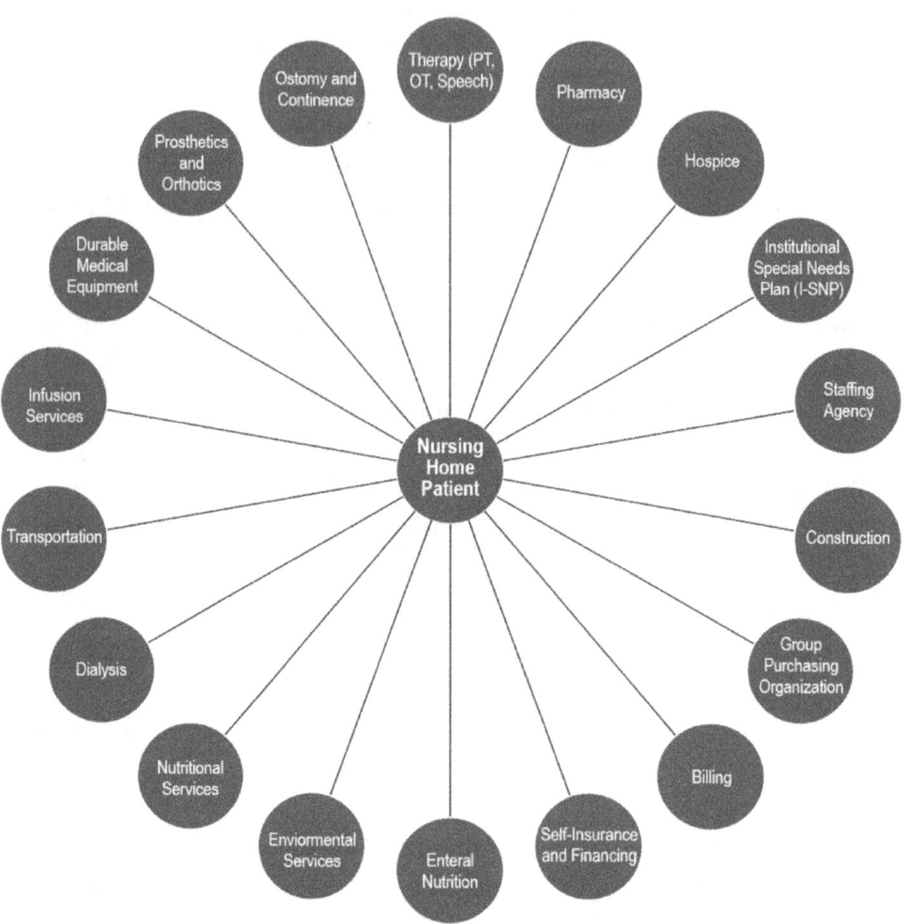

Source: Dave Devereaux

One page, made of circles and lines, depicting a Ferris wheel or Tinkertoy assembly—can be a nursing home company's *entire* strategic business plan.

Without patients, and a constant flow of them—*this machinery breaks.*

Managing the Fuel Supply

Ignore the byzantine legal structures and the gyrations exhibited by owners and executives when demanding these companies be treated as discrete entities. Instead, watch their behaviors and *follow the money.*

While pleading poverty about unsatisfactory taxpayer funding, or seeking increased protection from inflation, regulation, litigation, and legislation, owners and executives stoke an entirely different narrative.

Meetings and conversations usually begin with:

"We've started a new company."

"We're in a new JV (joint venture)." Or,

"We've reached an arrangement with a new strategic partner ..."

Almost immediately, *this* becomes the shiny new thing. Like a teenage infatuation, it's beautiful, flawless, perfect.

These shiny new things frequently involve no risk, competition, or constructive attention to price, quality, compliance, or governance. Especially when it involves family and friends.

Displaced vendors and prior partners, and their knowledge of the company, players, and practices evaporates, replaced by cheerleaders.

Like most shiny new things, age, use, and even misuse results in scuffs, scars, dents, and sometimes—problems. Same with these related-party ancillary businesses. Whether it be a therapy company, pharmacy, hospice, or institutional special needs plan (I-SNP), acne invades beauty, wrinkles appear, and what was once found to be perfect is no longer.

Nursing home administrators or directors of nursing will recount their miseries in changing pharmacy providers, for example. When involving a shiny new thing, or newly-created related-party business, even more so.

I witnessed one—switching from an incumbent pharmacy to a related-party business—in which the integration schedule accelerated to the point where multiple nursing homes—transitioning on a Saturday—suffered medication shortages, delivery delays, and electronic charting access barriers.

When reaching out to this new pharmacy's home and regional offices for help … *no one was home.*

This out-of-state pharmacy's leadership, the very architects of this ingenious plan, who were paid to support transitioning homes, were AWOL. Email, text, and phone call traffic recurred on subsequent Saturdays, and additional homes had similar experiences.

While the machinery's Ferris wheel or Tinkertoy assembly is common, it's very uncommon for related-party companies to have the infrastructure befitting of a real company, specifically in quality assurance, governance, and compliance.

As a ManCo executive, I can attest to organizing and overseeing efforts—using internal and external resources—to audit, examine, recommend improvement, and repeat these processes in areas involving coverage, eligibility, delivery, and propriety of care delivered to patients.

Granted, responsibility for some of these efforts rested with the nursing homes as a condition of licensure and payor contracting. Nevertheless, the total absence of these business fundamentals by related-party service providers, paid to touch and treat patients, was remarkable.

When discussing the absence of these fundamentals with leaders of these businesses, their eyes often glazed over, with an *"IDKWTF you are talking about"* stare coming back at me.

ᔓ

When things go wrong with shiny new things, cheerleading owners, investors, and executives of these *machinery* parts won't behave as if these businesses are discrete entities.

Ignoring resident rights, questions abound like, "Why aren't *we* (the related-party ancillary business) getting every (nursing home) patient?"

Or declarations will be launched, involving this specific sentence:

"We're getting far less than our *unfair share.*"

Having attended *thousands* of core business review meetings involving nursing homes, there were *hundreds* of occasions when questions asked of related-party ancillary company representatives, such as a rehabilitation company (or provider of physical, occupational, and speech therapy) involved responses like this:

"Our numbers are down, but the problem is the nursing home isn't admitting good patients."

Right.

Occasionally, an ancillary company representative, absent from a business review, opted to reach out privately. These phone conversations are memorable. This was one experience:

Hospice Salesperson: "Dave, I'd like to talk to you about what's going on in Region 4."

Me: "OK, what's on your mind?"

Hospice Salesperson: "Our volume is low. We're getting far less than our share."

Me: "OK, what does that mean?"

Hospice Salesperson: "We should be getting every hospice referral from these buildings!"

Me: "And you aren't, correct?"

Hospice Salesperson: "No, and I'd like to see what you can do about it."

Me: "Sounds like someone is beating you in this market. When you spoke to the administrators of these nursing homes, what did they tell you?"

Hospice Salesperson: (no audible sound)

Me: "OK, when you spoke to the director of operations or VP, what did they tell you?"

Hospice Salesperson: "I figured you could help me with this."

Me: "I just did."

When hospice representatives attended meetings and were asked by company leadership about shortfalls to revenue or census goals, this was a commonly-heard refrain:

"We're light right now, but it will pick up. There just aren't enough nursing home patients dying right now."

I'll not throw any more shade at rehab professionals or hospice workers. They play a vital role in taking care of people, and their services are desired and essential.

But their value doesn't make these experiences any less real.

Remarks like "admitting the wrong patients" or "aren't enough nursing home patients dying" can become very dangerous when said in front of a wrong-minded, misguided, or comparatively "poor" person of power within the machinery.

Why? Because these people consider these remarks to indicate *real problems*, requiring *real solutions*.

Candidly, they are neither. Nevertheless, it didn't stop people from creating problems out of thin air, expecting remedies that would be stupid—and could be harmful.

Superiors have given me instructions like, "You guys (nursing homes) need to admit better patients and be a better business partner" and asked questions like, "When will we see more patients be at their end-of-life point?"

These are situations where the best possible answer to the inquiring superior is:

"I don't know. Let me get back to you on this."

And wish that follow-up questions aren't asked or someone—in their zeal to seek favor—doesn't propose a wrong-minded or misguided solution that continues exhibiting blindness to patients as people.

Until it happens, again.

ᔓᔕ

This dynamic—involving related-party businesses—is true in assembly of companies whose business plan is to acquire or assemble parts of the *machinery*, and sit—watching the daily patient activity within nursing homes in the same way a degenerate gambler looks at their daily racing sheet to learn where *their* winning horses—I mean, new patients—are coming from.

Owners, as self-appointed managers—or appointed, pliable family members (or BFFs) serving as lead representatives of these various businesses—exhibit a near instant disregard for their former core businesses, routinely succumbing to incisive remarks made by reps of shiny new thing(s), embracing the narrative of *The nursing home is the problem.*

And sometimes, it is. Only sometimes.

This tension was fully displayed when attending meetings involving I-SNPs, where the profitability of the plan and the nursing home is influenced by keeping nursing home patients *out* of the hospital and *away* from the therapy (PT, OT, Speech) departments.

Many times, I found it hard to figure out exactly *who* the client was.

As I-SNP profitability depends on the number of covered patients (by the plan), and the productivity of the nurse practitioner assigned to the home to meet and treat covered patients, any drop in covered patients, or increase in the number of covered patients hospitalized, was viewed by stakeholders as a very bad thing.

For the nursing home, less covered patients and increased hospitalizations or treatments jeopardized incentive payments the home could receive from the plan.

Among those financially rewarded from this feature of the *machinery*, when things didn't go well, *the nursing home was the problem.*

And when the nursing home wasn't the problem, *the patient was the problem.*

I've witnessed conclusions drawn by executives and investors whose personal and work histories involved never touching a nursing home patient, who'd have required hospitalization if another person's poop, pee, puke, or blood touched them.

Fascinatingly, these people practiced their own versions of armchair medicine—all on behalf of the *machinery*.

Better Than WD-40

"We direct bill."

This is the irresistible sales strategy of companies just outside the machinery. The nursing home doesn't have to pay a penny. Let the company in, and they'll handle everything.

For decades, this oft-repeated sentence was the only thing needed for nursing homes to vote YES!

Admittedly, this simple, seductive approach is incredibly tempting. Always has been, and always will be. Like Medicare Advantage and potential enrollees. Sign here, and you'll pay *nothing*.

Nursing homes, in enterprises with related-party businesses, avoid temptation, as their relationships are assigned. Assignments can also include other businesses—owned and run by friends.

Like gears in an even larger machine, financial dialysis of nursing home patients goes far beyond one company—or group of companies under the same ownership structure. In this model, illustrated below, the possibilities for expanded patient dialyzing are considerable.

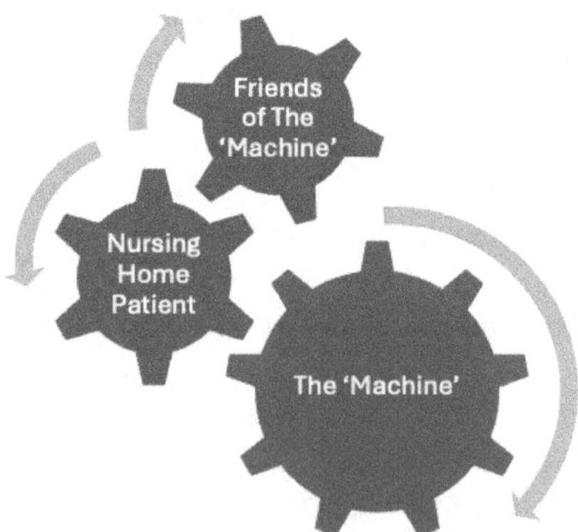

Before going further on this topic, here's a fact that shouldn't be surprising: It's not hard to rip off Medicare or Medicaid.

It happens in healthcare every minute, daily. A quick browser search unearths details of fraud and abuse involving physicians, pharmacies, COVID testing agencies, DME providers … and nursing homes too.

It's easy.

This first story involves a company and their "We direct bill" sales strategy. In the ostomy and continence business, it supplied nursing homes with products for patients suffering from incontinence of bowel, bladder, or both.

New and ambitious, and friends with company ownership, they sought a foothold into the nursing home company I worked for. Occasionally, representatives from this group visited the company's office, calling on the chief nursing officer, making presentations to nursing field leadership and knocking themselves out in an effort to *get in*.

Yet for all this effort, this hadn't happened. I first met this group—and its team—at a dinner they hosted. During dessert, a deck of PowerPoint slides followed, with this message:

"We direct bill. Your patients can get hundreds of catheters per month, free … if they need 'em."

Attendees didn't need to attend medical school to know that each of our nursing home patients had only *one* urethra, and they didn't self-catheterize. As a provider, we wanted to have catheters in as *few* patients as possible, and *only* when medically necessary.

I asked two questions:

- Who's your company's medical director?
- What's your company's compliance program?

Their response:

"We don't need a medical director or compliance program. We have this lady, and she's great. I'd love for you to meet her. She and her team fill out the Certificates of Medical Necessity for all the patients. If we do something wrong, Medicare won't pay … that's it."

My thought—this company might be a pizza shop with a Medicare provider number. And it doesn't sell pizza.

Because of their relationship with my employer, rules of engagement dictated that they were given one final chance to demonstrate their wares.

So, they were. We asked them to revisit in thirty days, with a medical director and compliance program in tow, or it would be the last time we spoke about any sort of business arrangement.

Thirty days later, the rep returned, presenting to a group routinely assembled to vet and credential vendors and service providers.

The two questions from the previous meeting were repeated. The answers were: *"We don't have a medical director,"* even at a contracted level of a few hours a month; and the same to any semblance of a compliance program.

This wasn't a waste of time and energy. It did, however, throw sand into the machinery's gears.

ꙮ

Treasure hunts like this continue. Still.

This is a recent, unedited LinkedIn message from a sender identified as a "CPA, licensed nursing home administrator and health care financial turnaround consultant."

Hi Dave,

FREE SUPPLIES!
Did you know you could receive the following supplies for FREE ...

Ostomy supplies
Wound Care supplies
Diabetic shoes
Urological/Catheter supplies

Enteral feeding supplies (tube feed)
Lymphedema supplies
Some Negative Pressure Equipment

For a qualifying resident, you just need a Medicare Part B biller/supplier who will handle it all for you!

I've attached an example of how much one of my healthcare clients is saving ($156K per year!)

Make sure you're not leaving money on the table!

IT'S LIKE FREE MONEY and a no-brainer way to immediately improve your profit margin! ? I am happy to refer you to a great Part B vendor if you need one!

Have a wonderful Holiday!

God bless,
Bonnie (fictitious name)

Another pizza shop (maybe) with a Medicare provider number, and an e-commerce campaign. Wonder how this "CPA, licensed nursing home administrator and healthcare financial turnaround consultant" gets paid? By a gear in a patient financial dialysis machine—somewhere. Maybe?

Total Breakdowns

When shiny new things become dull, or *machinery* parts and gears don't *maximize* financial output, people with the most to gain will begin spinning out.

At one company, whose core strategy was financially dialyzing each patient, an owner—who managed multiple related-party companies—entered my office, breaking up a separate meeting already in progress.

Dazed, and doing his best imitation of the pee-pee dance, he looked around, whimpering: "Dave, I need to cancel this afternoon's meeting. I'm wearing two hats today and just don't have the time." Watching him exit the office, chin to chest, I wondered when he had acquired a second head to satisfy his additional hat.

With some recovery time, shot callers' spirits become resurrected, resuming their hunt for shiny new things to put into the *machinery*, growing additional heads for hats to rest upon, further diluting their attention from traditional core businesses—or redefining *the core* as their related-party ancillary companies—and recharging their proverbial battery packs, resuming *financial dialysis* on nursing home patients.

Some recoveries are protracted. Especially when the nursing home(s) patient census declines. When this occurs, *machinery* custodians will become manic in attempting to maximize output.

Knowing that it all starts with input—nursing home patients—you might hear:

"We'll take anything! Even Medicaid!"

Without nursing home patients, and a constant flow of them, this *machinery* breaks.

Some exceed this clarion call. Nursing home executives—demanding more patients to feed their machinery, seeking instant gratification or lifestyle sustenance, or managing an allergy to competition—can behave abhorrently. With a partner—or partners—they can be downright despicable.

These behaviors, historically attributed to "lone wolves" or "bad actors," have evolved from isolated incidents to raising eyebrows and questions.

In an August 30, 2025, *McKnight's* editorial, "Hoping for God's Grace is a Dangerous Business Strategy," John O'Connor—a veteran opinionator and industry treasure—writes about behaviors within the industry and the ability to "do the right thing."

Two questions O'Connor raises about the scope and depth of law enforcement investigations—and sanctions—of OpCos, PropCos, and ManCos:

- Is the problem really just a few bad apples?
- Or is it something deeper, that too many are hoping (Attorneys General and friends) won't come knocking?[56]

While these questions get sorted, I'll share two instances where the pursuit of additional nursing home patients intersected with incredibly bad behavior.

This first story cites a June 28, 2023, Becker's Hospital Review article, "California Nursing Home to Pay $3.8M for Physician Referral Scheme."

As reported:

> From 2009 through 2019, Riverside, Calif.-based Alta Vista Healthcare & Wellness Centre and its management company, Los Angeles-based Rockport Healthcare Services, gave certain physicians extravagant gifts and paid them monthly stipends of $2,500 to $4,000 for their services as medical directors. At least one purpose of the gifts *was to entice physicians to refer patients* (emphasis added) to Alta Vista, according to a June 21 Justice Department news release. This resulted in false claims to Medicare and California's Medicaid programs.[57]

This behavior resulted in Alta Vista and Rockport being fined over $3.2 million by the Feds, and almost $600,000 by the State of California.[58]

Enticing physicians to refer patients sounds a lot like getting paid to help feed the *machinery*.

Another publication, helped define *gifts*. In its June 21, 2023, article, "California nursing facility agrees to pay $3.8 million for alleged kickbacks to doctors," *USA Today* reported "expensive dinners for physicians and their spouses, golf trips, limousine rides, massages, e-reader tablets, and gift cards up to $1,000."[59]

Like the definition of "poor" shared earlier, what constitutes "expensive" is equally relative. Then again—it doesn't really matter. The behavior, however, does.

And these shenanigans were separate from the nearly *$30–50,000* this nursing home and their company paid annually for medical direction.[60] Since the articles reference physicians (plural), it's hard to determine just how much money was coming out of this home—and company—*to pay doctors hired to feed the machine.*

Alta Vista is a ninety-nine bed nursing home.[61] Their 2025 web page is sparse. Their site is completely devoid of ***any*** leadership identification—by face, name, or title.[62]

You won't find a website or any publicly available, company produced information about Rockport Healthcare Services. You'll have to scour LinkedIn, Indeed, Facebook, industry publications, and www.oig.hhs.gov to find *anything*. It doesn't appear that they want to be found.

Some important work, done by *The Sacramento Bee*, as well as BriusWatch.org focuses specifically on another company—Brius Healthcare.[63] Interestingly, Brius Healthcare also has no web presence, though the information found on BriusWatch helps connect Alta Vista—the nursing home—with this company.[64]

Where Rockport fits—today—is elusive. Maybe that's how Alta Vista's owners like it. It looks like Brius is the successor to Rockport, though stating definitively would require additional information.

Retrospectively, I wonder if Alta Vista and the invisibles affiliated with Rockport Healthcare (or Brius, maybe) considered all this worth it.

Guess it depends on understanding their priorities and incentives. Plus additional information indicating PropCo, ManCo, and any other Cos like those illustrated in the grids and graphics shared within this chapter. Something this intentionally complex would rapidly become simpler.

But here's a question for the agencies that went after this nursing home:

Did the Department of Justice and the State of California follow the money, and take back any ill-gotten gains—like the revenue received by related-party ancillary companies that Rockport Healthcare Services (or related-party owners) required Alta Vista to use—when treating patients referred and secured through these bribes and kickbacks?

There's silence on this item. If take-backs weren't pursued, maybe the players looked at $3.8 million in penalties as a price worth paying—to keep their *machinery* running.

Embarrassingly, Alta Vista–Rockport isn't a stand-alone example of incredibly bad behavior. These next misfires, occurring on the opposite side of the nation, might be considered *one-upmanship*.

ꟼ

In April 2019, the exploits of Philip Esformes, a South Florida nursing home owner, surpassed Alta Vista–Rockport's shenanigans, leaving the industry with a permanent black eye.

Candidly, this is gratuitous imagery.

Considered to be the "largest health care fraud scheme ever charged by the U.S. Department of Justice," the price tag on Esformes' fraudulent behavior reached $1.3 billion.[65] In achieving this distinction, Esformes was convicted of:[66]

- one count of conspiracy to defraud the United States
- two counts of receipt of kickbacks in connection with a federal health care program
- four counts of payment of kickbacks in connection with a federal health care program
- one count of conspiracy to commit money laundering
- nine counts of money laundering, two counts of conspiracy to commit federal program bribery
- one count of obstruction of justice

All told, twenty criminal counts. The only thing missing? A partridge in a pear tree.

In the process, Esformes pocketed an estimated $37 million—for himself.[67]

Esformes and his late father Morris, "an Orthodox rabbi and founder of the family business," had owned and operated nursing homes and assisted living facilities in Chicago, Missouri, and Florida.[68]

Here's a highlight reel, covering 1998 to 2016:

- Esformes paid cash to a physician's assistant and a hospital administrator for "recycled patients" and illegal kickbacks to doctors to ***refer patients*** to his homes.[69]
- Drug addicts, some of whom didn't require nursing home care, were provided opioids without a physician's order, to entice them to stay at Esformes' facilities.[70]
- A coconspirator stated that he referred patients to Esformes whether they needed services or not, paying kickbacks to Esformes in return for Esformes referring patients to use the coconspirators' ancillary businesses—*pharmacy, home healthcare and other services.* Esformes accepted kickbacks from other providers who sought access to Esformes' patients to bill Medicare for services that were unnecessary or fake.[71]
- At least one payment of $5,000 was made to Florida regulators at the Agency for Health Care Administration to provide advance information about unannounced health inspections to Esformes' facilities so that Esformes could falsify records in advance of agency inspection visits.[72]
- In 2015, Esformes plotted to help one of his coconspirators leave Florida for Israel to avoid trial by providing an "empty seat", a plot caught on tape by the Feds due to a coconspirator wearing a wire.[73]
- Around the time of his indictments, a federal judge ordered Esformes to return money wrongly transferred to his

father, residing in Chicago, in a failed attempt to protect his assets.[74]

- Several coconspirators pled guilty and cooperated with federal prosecutors, including some who testified against Esformes.[75]

This illustrates the lengths that nursing home owners and executives have taken to keep their *machines* from breaking. And not be "poor"—relative to others.

ᔓ

It is difficult—in both instances—to understand the motivation.

Why'd they do it? Here are a few questions in search of the *Why*:

- Because they needed a constant flow of patients to sustain the ancillary companies within the *machinery* (related-party or friends providing kickbacks)?
- Because the grip of anticompetitive behavior was so ingrained—and heretofore rewarded—that competing straight-up for the trust of patients and families was just too hard?

Or ...

- Because the sense of entitlement—to lifestyle sustenance—was so overpowering, that regardless of cost—rules applied only to others, but not to "us"?

Maybe, it was all of the above. And putting patients through these versions of financial dialysis was overwhelmingly irresistible.

What raises these questions? We'll complete this chapter by recapping how Esformes's ill-gotten gains were used.

- Real estate properties in Miami Beach, Chicago, and Los Angeles, and unencumbered assets (debt-free) worth $79 million[76]
- A LaFerrari Aperta sports car[77]
- A Greubel Forsey watch, estimated to be worth $360,000[78]
- $400,000 paid to Rick Singer, the man at the center of the college bribery scandal, Operation Varsity Blues, to "slip his daughter into USC as a fake soccer player and fix his son's college entrance exam"[79]
- $300,000 paid to University of Pennsylvania basketball coach Jerome Allen, who testified that he received cash and wire transfers to get Esformes's son on the UPenn basketball team and into the Wharton School of Business[80]
- $114,000 paid to Martin Fox, a Texas sports coach and convicted co-conspirator of Singer, "to provide one-on-one basketball coaching" for his son[81]
- Airfare and chauffeured limousines for escorts' travel to Orlando, Florida for liaisons with Esformes at the Ritz-Carlton Hotel[82]

The razzle-dazzle of OpCo, PropCo, and ManCo is intentional. This is to make you look, and desperately try to figure out who does what for whom, and why. Knowing this exists—and why—matters.

What matters more is how the patient fits inside this machinery, the behaviors of those with most to gain, and … *following the money.*

WHAT YOU CAN DO

Ask Questions About:

- Which "Co" people work for?
- Which "Co" is responsible, for what, and how does someone know?
- Relationships with related-party ancillary companies.
- Service providers that directly bill Medicare and other insurers.
- Common ownership—in any combination of businesses.

Look for:

- Website information on the "Co." If it doesn't exist, red flags are flying.
- Information on related-party companies. If absent, they might be a pizza shop.

Listen to What People Say:

- How do people identify "the owner(s)"?
- What does the word "We" mean? It's an indicator of behavior, which may differ from how "Co" is portrayed ... *on paper*.

V

NURSING HOMES STRUGGLE TO PASS AN OPEN BOOK TEST

Imagine ... on the first day of school—every year and grade—you needed only one book for the school year. Every test for the entire year is based on this book, with all tests open book.

Imagine ... your grades—in the second year. Better than the first? Or would you coast into a lesser grade?

Testing Eligibility

Nursing homes are licensed by their states. Without one, they're out of business.

Licenses come with numerous requirements, ranging from the building's internal temperature to patient care delivery. Requirements evolve. As they do, it's the nursing home's job to remain up-to-date and compliant.

Very few nursing homes are licensed as private-only, where patients pay for services in cash or non-taxpayer-funded payment. These homes are overseen by their respective states, and while compliance with licensing regulations is challenging, it pales in comparison to most nursing homes nationally.

All other nursing homes will contract with the federal and state governments, becoming a participating (or certified) provider in Medicare and Medicaid, receiving taxpayer-funded payment for patient services.

These homes are required to comply with state licensure requirements *and* their Medicare and Medicaid provider agreements. The State conducts a *survey* of the home, and determines its compliance.

This survey is the *open book test*.

States share survey results with their federal counterparts, the Centers for Medicare and Medicaid Services (CMS) Regional Office. Nursing homes are assigned a CMS Regional Office (RO), determined by its location. ROs accept or reject the findings of the State's survey findings.

When the State and CMS agree, survey results are issued to the home, with findings and timetables for corrective action.

The Book

On CMS's website, its *State Operations Manual* is found under *Regulations and Guidance*. This manual, historically referred to as the "Watermelon Book," due to its distinctive red color, is the ***900+*** page tome of definitions, interpretive guidelines, procedures, and potential citations used by nursing homes—and surveyors—in determining regulatory compliance.[83]

The Book is shared with nursing homes to eliminate secrets about the What, How, and Why requirements are reviewed. While things change daily within a nursing home, the Watermelon Book rarely does—and homes are informed months or years in advance.

Why Good Grades Matter

Solid and improving grades, year after year should be easy. Right? *Book and test don't change. Test is always open book.*

Some nursing homes achieve outstanding survey results, reflecting solid and improving grades. Others—*don't*.

Why?

Because it's hard work. And it's easier to coast.

A quick aside—this chapter covers many areas regarding nursing home compliance and performance, yet excludes any statistical comparisons or analyses in these areas. If you're interested in a nursing home's single or multiyear survey performance history, go to www.medicare.gov. You can drill down on the number, type, and intensity of deficiencies a nursing home has earned in previous surveys.[84]

Let's compare this process to another regulated industry—restaurants. The score of its last health and sanitation inspection is usually a letter-graded card posted in their window, or a numeric rating near the cashier's station. Ratings or scores influence the dining decision—or not.

Some people don't care. Any restaurant could have a bad day. Most restaurant health inspections are just that—a day. Usually a few hours.

Surveys are substantially different, lasting numerous *days*, with several subject-matter experts participating. Some surveyors have prior nursing home work experience, which they'd rate from excellent to terrible. Others have none. Survey teams will include trainees, eager to show their wares to superiors. Surveys can last weeks with teams of ten-plus people simultaneously examining a home.

Surveys don't end after surveyors leave for the day. Until they return, the home's leadership reviews notes of observations, working to assure that the issues noted aren't repeated. Repeat issues involving individual patients, individual workers, or specific departments usually spell unpleasant survey outcomes.

Intense? *Yes*.

Necessary? Probably.

Considering what a nursing home does and the responsibilities that homes and surveyors have to patients and taxpayers, surveys shouldn't be a one-day deal. This is complex, important work, demanding time and a team of people to do it.

ᔕ

Nursing home caregivers, department heads, administrators, and owners cite the state survey process as one of the greatest hardships in their working experience.

This is understandable. Surveys are grueling. Nevertheless—*they're not new.*

Nursing home workers also remark that surveys *scare the living hell* out of some people. On its face, surveys shouldn't be scary. It's an open book test.

What's scary, however, is guessing which questions will be asked, and to whom they'll be directed. It's scary not knowing when a survey will occur. The state survey agency doesn't make an appointment.

They'll show up anytime, unannounced, investigating complaints filed against the home, or issues the home self-reports under its requirements as a mandatory reporter. Surveys can occur on weekends. This requires the nursing home to be in a constant state of readiness.

Stakes are high with surveys. Enforcement for poor performance can be expensive and painful.

Civil money penalties (CMPs)—translation: fines—can accompany deficiencies, totaling five, six, or seven figures. I've seen state survey agencies and CMS levy CMPs totaling $50,000 and more for citations that ranged from legitimate to total BS.

Nursing homes have limited leverage in disputing these decisions and penalties, as these agencies are both contractor and payor.

Fighting back is expensive, can burn bridges, and risks other company homes as payback candidates in future surveys. Many times, I picked the path of least resistance, paying the fine timely, taking the 35 percent discount offered for undisputed payment, and working to avoid repeating these deficiencies.

Other industries may treat a $50,000 fine as the cost of doing business. For a nursing home, this is the salary equivalent of a nurse, or almost two certified nursing assistants. Several hundred thousand dollar CMPs threaten a home's present and future operations.

Homes can be denied payment for new admissions when certain deficiencies are repeated in successive surveys or deemed uncorrected. This prohibition quickly results in six-figure losses in revenue, especially for nursing homes reliant on short-stay medical and rehabilitation patients.

When a state loses trust in a nursing home's leadership, they may direct a plan of correction to address deficiencies, thus eliminating the home's ability to create an action plan, or mandate an appointed quality monitor to oversee what occurs within the home.

Exceptionally poor survey performance or failing to correct deficiencies over a defined period can result in revocation of a home's Medicare and Medicaid certification. Homes are then forced into a cooling-off period, taxpayer-funded governmental payments dry up, and the home is required to pass a recertification survey for participation and payment restoration.

Finally, they can suffer what's referred to as the *death penalty*, or license termination, which requires transferring patients to other locations and a step into hell for people affiliated with the nursing home.

Long before a nursing home reaches license termination, *the license of the home's nursing home administrator* can be jeopardized—including revocation.

I've visited, advised, operated, or overseen nearly one thousand nursing homes across the country—and witnessed the impact of every one of these enforcement actions.

For nursing home companies with multiple locations in a region or state, it's routine for surveyors to share survey findings for homes under common ownership or brand, examining patterns in organization, behavior, resources, and governance. The reputation of a company is influenced by the lowest common denominators among its homes. Here's an example.

Years ago, I led a team of nurses and lawyers to examine the multiyear history of state survey performance for each of the company's nursing homes.

The average number of deficiencies for this nursing home portfolio was greater than ten, ranging from zero to thirty-plus. Several of the homes had thousands of dollars in fines and penalties during the sample period.

This project's purpose was to determine:

- The company's most frequently cited deficiencies
- The root causes of these deficiencies—structural, indicating design flaws with the company's approach; or executional, indicating flaws in day-to-day survey management by individual nursing homes
- Adjustments—structural, strategic, or tactical—to reduce the deficiencies incurred, CMPs paid, and overall risk through improved state survey performance

This scope of work involved us each reviewing every home's statement of deficiencies over a three-year period. We found lowest common denominators in knowing the patient, building patient relationships, service quality, technique breaches, and governance.

This exposed structural flaws. Some areas required improved messaging, while others required state-specific adjustments or refinements to meet varying guidelines by location.

Deficiencies due to execution in survey management were twice the rate of structural flaws, falling into the following categories:

- People or things that should've been clean ... weren't.
- Things that should've been thrown out or returned ... weren't.
- Issues that should've been known ... weren't.

Most homes had outsourced housekeeping, laundry, dining, and therapy services to third-party providers. In too many cases, the nursing home's administrator had ceded responsibility for departmental oversight and quality management to the provider representative.

Compared to other elements influencing survey performance, these weren't hard to remedy. It just took people committed to doing it.

ꟹ

Last, nursing home owners, executives, administrators, and trade association representatives want surveyors to be *more collaborative, or more collegial*, mirroring the relationship homes have with the Joint Commission, formerly known as the Joint Commission on Accreditation of Healthcare Organizations (JCAHO), a nongovernmental agency.

Unaffiliated with licensure and certification, nursing homes *elect to pay* the Joint Commission to survey—with advanced notice—issue findings, and determine accreditation for a defined period.[85]

This desired collaboration presumes that providers and regulators share the same goal—achieving what is best for the patient.

Sound reasonable? Provider representatives think so.

OK. Let's try to add some texture to this topic and apply what is known:

Nursing homes are paid to take an open book test, and the answers are available to all the relevant questions.

They're paid with taxpayer money to take this test.

As a student, would you ask your parent, or teacher, to help you take this open book test?

It appears this is what some nursing home leaders want. Why? Because the work required is hard. And they want someone else to help them do it.

I've never been employed by a state survey agency. Presuming what goes on inside this agency isn't something I'll do.

My impressions are based on time spent with surveyors, team leaders, supervisors, and chiefs of state survey agencies and departments of health, and their equivalents on the federal side—including CMS, the Office of Inspector General, and Department of Justice.

I've learned that regulators are aware of the demands and challenges incumbent on a nursing home and are open-minded to discuss work to improve an individual nursing home or nursing home company.

I've invited—and welcomed—agency representatives to attend and participate in nursing home and company meetings, providing education in areas involving the Watermelon Book, interpretive guidelines, and enforcement.

During the early 2000s, for example, state licensure guidelines were found to have structural gaps when surveying nursing homes with areas dedicated to caring for patients with Alzheimer's disease and related memory disorders.

Rather than taking a dogmatic approach to existing regulations, departments of health in *two* states examined guidelines created by the nursing home company that employed me, later incorporating these guidelines into separate state survey applications for nursing homes with this programming.

Under certain circumstances, collaboration was real.

At the same time, there was a complete understanding of these agencies' roles, which was to survey and certify nursing homes, recommending enforcement when necessary. That's it. And really, how it should be.

Nursing homes (and companies) seeking a collaborative effort in achieving or maintaining survey excellence have multiple options available, *beyond* the state survey agency. Many homes routinely have access to nursing consultants, highly skilled people providing expert technical assistance across a broad spectrum of areas.-

Homes without this consultation have no barriers to adding this dimension. Qualified, experienced people are available to assist. When demand exceeds an individual consultant's capacity, firms providing expanded services are available.

The Test

Nursing home administrators, directors of nursing, and departmental leaders experience *butterflies* before, and during, a survey. Like athletes before a season opener, students before their exams, and performing artists before their recitals.

Butterflies are healthy. My experience, shared with nursing home leaders for years, is that they create focus and acceptance of outcomes … if you've prepared well.

Execution flaws are expected during surveys. People make mistakes under direct observation.

Imagine someone observing your *every* move while caring for someone. Administering medications. Preparing meals. That's what a survey is like for nursing home workers, leadership, and executives. Imagine doing this while being asked by an untrusted stranger:

"Can you tell me what you're doing?"

"Can you tell me why you're doing it this way?"

"Can you tell me who taught you to do it this way?"

"Can you tell me what the policy and procedure is for what you're doing?"

This is hard. People who've been through a nursing home survey will say *it is miserable*. How can this be? It's an open book test. The answers are known! Yes. The book and test are static. But everything else is dynamic.

Nursing homes' patient populations change daily. In minutes, a patient's condition or mood can change. In a phone call, physician orders and medications can change. By shift, nursing home employees can change. By survey, surveying team members can change.

These dynamics disrupt a nursing home's flow, adding difficulty to *acing* the open book test.

Survey preparedness is never accidental. The nursing home and its owners must be invested, individually and collectively. This investment isn't a one-and-done. It's required daily. When committed to this process-based investment, results become consistently excellent.

Process-based investment yields the highest returns through:

- **Rounding.** Walking the home's interior and exterior, independently or with any combination of people. Looking up, down, left, and right. Observing. Taking notes. Communicating action items to teammates. Following up until satisfied. Keeping little problems little.
- **Start-up and wrap-up sessions**. Assembling leadership at the beginning and ending of each day to communicate expected and actual developments and status updates on critical issues.
- **Patient assessment.** Knowing each patient's condition—at and after admission, and the subtle and remarkable changes—as they occur.
- **Care planning.** Effectively planning the goals and approaches to delivering care based on patient condition, revisiting plans with changing care needs.
- **Developing people.** Making each other smarter daily. Providing encouragement, refining techniques, and building confidence. Same as what occurs at halftime in a football or basketball game, or between innings in baseball. Investing minutes daily is powerfully effective when compounded over time.
- **Quality assurance and process improvement.** Remaining honest about the home's work. Measuring results and outcomes over time. Comparing to increasingly ambitious goals and metrics, without enabling or excusing shortfalls.
- **Simulated surveys.** a.k.a. pre-survey, or mock survey. Applying rigor to be tougher than a State survey. Using

the Watermelon Book *and* the nursing home's policies, procedures, and guidelines in developing corrective action plans. Following up relentlessly.

Homes with consistently excellent surveys do these things. Shortcuts might satisfy a single survey cycle, though time and dynamism eventually catches up to the home, delivering a healthy dose of pain.

Test Takers

While a nursing home prepares for a survey, individual readiness and execution during the survey can't be underestimated. Like in team sports, there are occasions when individual performance matters.

Prepared, confident people excel during surveys. Their daily work approach and technique mirrors every other. For them, surveys aren't hard. They're irritating.

People who like shortcuts, are new to the work or role, identify English as their second language—don't get butterflies. These employees are terrified. Because they're unprepared. Surveys can leave lifelong scars on their psyche. These scars result from execution errors, directly tracing back to the "Three P's—Piss. Poor. Preparation."

Surveyor attention forces these execution errors, which fall into the following categories:

- **Awareness.** People don't know what they are supposed to know, or where to be, and might not know that they don't know what they are supposed to know.
- **Organization.** People might know what they are supposed to do yet don't do it at the right place or time.
- **Communication.** People don't tell each other what needs to be done, what they have done, or what is happening.

- **Discipline.** People know what to do, where and when to do it, and simply don't do it.
- **Team play.** People decide that nothing is their job, or everything is their job, instead of doing their own job and helping when possible.

Why does this happen?
It's hard to get everything consistently right, with excellence.

Who's Being Tested?

Tell me, who is responsible for scarring these unprepared people? Surveyors? The individual? The nursing home?

I've always believed that responsibility for employee execution errors and the resultant scar tissue rests with the nursing home's *leadership*. Surveys are open book tests. Answer keys are available.

Nursing home leaders are sometimes unprepared. I've known administrators to bury themselves in their offices during surveys, forfeiting oversight to direct reports, and relinquishing ownership of survey results.

People loathe to owning survey preparation or execution errors, and under fire during surveyor interviews, might say, "This is how the company makes us do it."

Though I've read this in reports, I can't ever recall it accompanying a survey with five or fewer deficiencies.

In instances where nursing home ownership or executive leadership demonstrates a historical reluctance, ambivalence, or indifference toward the investments referenced earlier, their responsibility supersedes nursing home leadership.

I've known owners and executives whose survey philosophy was, *When they cite it, we will fix it.*

Philosophical litmus tests often involve a home's physical plant or large and immovable equipment requiring repair, maintenance, or replacement—or work involving four- to five-figure expenditures. Required remedies are deferred, with bets made on the nursing home's—and nursing home administrator's—licenses.

My favorite example is a leaky roof. Roof leaks range from what you'd see at home, remedied by a pot on the floor, to a "natural skylight," or a *big* hole in the roof and ceiling.

Want a rainforest effect in a nursing home? Deferring maintenance or repair on a small roof leak will do it. Like a house plant, all it needs is water.

Want to give an owner a seizure? Request that a leaky roof be fixed correctly. Some will totally freak out.

The predictable response to this request? "Use vinyl garbage containers. Put 'em out and store 'em away when it isn't raining. If surveyors show up, put up clean ceiling tile. Leave 'em there until they're gone."

Nothing is off-limits when homes take the open book test. Washers, dryers, dishwashers, boilers, air handling and fire safety systems, and elevators must all pass muster.

During survey or not, work is harder when these items aren't in top working condition. To do the work that people are paid for, they need the right tools, all the time.

Like hospitals and hotels, homes deliver services where all elements involving patient and worker safety *should* be status quo.

There's a baseline expectation that patients are fed, bathed, clothed, weighed, transported, and cared for without negative consequences. This same expectation of safety applies to workers.

When these expectations aren't met, doubt spreads. Workers, patients, and families begin wondering whether the nursing home owner values their safety and the patients they serve.

This is dangerous territory. A diminished view about a home's value structure exposes the home to any curious response to a surveyor's question. Surveyors will explore managerial parsimony, ignorance, indifference, weakness, or fear, with the nursing home paying the price.

Missing equipment or supplies to meet baseline expectations indicate shortcuts, threatening patient or personal safety. This might be individual objects. Or vital parts of something bigger.

Instances when an elevator, for example, is out of commission for a day, weekend, or longer can pose serious issues. In homes with multiple functioning elevators, one disabled elevator car might be an inconvenience. When a nursing home has only one elevator, and it goes down, everything gets harder. Every risk heightens, including passing the open book test.

This is what a multistory nursing home experiences when this happens:

- Everyone *must* use the stairs. But not everyone *can* use the stairs.
- Deliveries *must* go up or down the stairs. Nursing home deliveries *can* be huge.
- Food carts *cannot* go up the stairs. Patient trays *must* go up the stairs one at a time (or two).
- Hot food becomes cold, and cold food becomes warm or hot.
- Medication delivery carts *cannot* go up the stairs.
- *The stairwells stink*. Dirty food trays and dirty laundry *must* travel to be washed.
- Patient transportation (to therapy, appointments, activities, dining) is altered or ceases.
- Patient admissions and discharges are extremely difficult.
- *911* calls involving patients can become dangerous.
- Someone always seems to get hurt. A trip, fall, sprained ankle, or worse occurs.

Though this isn't a comprehensive list, hard things become harder. Mistakes can be made, people can be hurt, and the likelihood of cleanly passing the test increasingly diminishes. Worker and visitor goodwill suffers as this inconvenience lengthens.

Patient risks and service interruptions are a gamble, the results of which might not be known for a while—maybe never if no one complains about it.

ᔕ

Pivoting to something smaller in scale, let's spotlight a home's dining department, where equipment deficits can be massively impactful. This department, including the home's kitchen operation, requires numerous pieces of small and large, fixed and movable equipment. Nursing homes can produce several hundred to a few thousand meals a day. Having enough equipment—that works—is critical.

While plates, bowls, cups, and utensils are essential for the department to run without disruption, shortages here don't send workers into the tailspin which makes everything harder. Bigger stuff does.

Replacement costs of things like dishwashers or stoves easily reaches four to five figures. Routine maintenance and respect for this equipment helps each to have a long and productive life.

An example is the home's walk-in cooler. Oftentimes, this box has a door that opens into the kitchen. Behind this door is a refrigerator, where racks hold cooked and uncooked food. Behind the refrigerator is another door and the freezer section.

Without properly functioning refrigerators and freezers, food can spoil. Unsafe food can cause food poisoning and even kill a nursing home patient.

Caring for afflicted patients who can't describe their symptoms is extremely challenging. Fever, vomiting, and diarrhea are symptoms of any number of illnesses. Working backward to determine potential causes is much easier when patients can communicate with an awareness of their own personal timeline.

Today, walk-ins use stainless and galvanized steel, aluminum, and insulation that can keep a beer cold for centuries. Models available today are remarkable. But doors, compressors, and floors age over time and wear out. This is visible to those paid to assess equipment needs.

Such equipment repairs cause sticker shock which leads to trade-offs—decision deferrals risk patient care, worker disenchantment, and compliance misfires.

Who's Being Tested?—Part Deux

We've all kicked the can down the road to stave off a big expense, or done half-baked repairs we know won't last to temporarily defer a big hit to our bank account.

Similarly, when learning that repairs will be large, unplanned, one-time operating expenses to a nursing home's monthly profit and loss statement, *rather than capitalized and depreciated over years*—decision-makers will sometimes play with short-term options and long-term solutions.

One-time operating expenses adversely impacting a quarterly or annual bonus might result in a desire to have the item replaced as a capital expense. This routinely requires reviews and approvals, and rejection or deferral. This burns time.

For cash-crunched or credit-poor companies, replacement may not be an option, leaving the operating expense as the path of least resistance. People don't like big-dollar surprises and will procrastinate before deciding.

We've all been there, but we don't care for tens, or hundreds, of people at home. This is the case in nursing homes, making cash, credit, and accounting treatment formidable realities when restoring equipment to full functionality ... *Quickly.*

ಌ

Company values—beyond accounting—broadly impact a nursing home's ability to pass the open book test. This next example spotlights something impacting our health every day ... and night.

I'm talking mattresses. A night on one not suited to you results in poor sleep, altered spinal alignment, or pain. Rising the next day might result in misery.

Long-term, they determine one's amount and quality of rest, influencing mood and stress levels. Unchecked stress can result in weight gain and hypertension, elevating heart disease and stroke risk—*among people who are not nursing home patients.*

Mattress integrity is essential in nursing homes. Sick and debilitated patients can spend most of their day in bed. Cracked or misshapen mattresses create risk for odors, infection, pain, and patient injury.

Some mattresses—even fresh from the box—can't satisfy a nursing home patient's needs. When they can't, things get harder—for patients and caregivers. Health risks become more prevalent for patients unable to rest or sleep, requiring additional caregiver intervention.

It's embarrassing to remember conversations within companies about mattress selection and quality, tripping over dollars to save pennies. Routinely, jousting matches ensued over this equipment, pitting Operations and Nursing leadership on one side, and Finance and Purchasing on the other.

Candidly, there were times I envisioned taking these colleagues to a nursing home, placing them in hand-cranked beds with the mattress they endorsed, pulling up the bedrails, and securing them in four-point restraints, returning the next morning to inquire about their night's sleep.

For decades, the nursing home standard was a spring-coiled, cloth mattress, protected by a plastic cover with a metal zipper or a rubber sheet. Later options included vinyl covering, improving infection control.

Options aside, mattresses are *hot*. Like sitting in a Naugahyde chair wearing shorts and a tank top. Sit in one for fifteen minutes and you will stick to the chair. Skin sticks to these mattresses. While a fitted sheet may separate patient and mattress, and the patient may be gowned or fully dressed, it is still *hot*.

Caregivers are the first line of defense in assessing mattress integrity, and this is evident the instant a bed is stripped. When mattress integrity isn't maintained, people work harder to compensate for the problem and patient care progress is sustained or improved. Or they don't, and patients suffer while their health degrades.

When basics like a comfortable mattress aren't provided, it sows distrust among hardworking nursing home staff.

This further threatens the home's credibility. If this cycle goes unbroken, workers break. If workers break, the nursing home breaks.

And can't possibly pass the open book test.

Shifting Values Helped Pass the Test

Company value structures, though seemingly intractable, can change to make things easier for nursing home patients and workers. This example involved a big investment, and was worth it.

I'm still talking mattresses.

At the time of a company-wide reorganization, its acquired pressure injury rate was 8 percent. This metric included many nursing homes that had significantly varying rates.

This singular indicator legitimizes impressions of nursing home leadership, caregiver competence and utilization, rehabilitation department effectiveness, commitment to patient care, quality assurance, and *equipment*.

Similarly, it raises questions about those hired to run, lead, and govern a company.

Through this reorganization, I was partnered with a newly appointed senior vice president of professional services, previously the company's vice president of risk management, whose new duties included enterprise-wide leadership and oversight of nursing and other functions influencing patient care.

She understood the company, its patient care performance, incidents and injuries resulting in litigation, and survey history. Her several years as a nursing home administrator were invaluable.

Among competing priorities during this change, driving down the company's acquired pressure injury rate was the largest, and most impactful to patients and workers.

Success meant a better experience for patients, improved survey outcomes, reduced litigation and associated costs, and improved nursing home and company performance through improved patient care.

Company-wide calculations estimated pressure injuries to cost *many* thousands per patient, depending on depth, size, duration, and treatment approach. When litigated, compensatory and punitive damages ranged from the mid-to-upper six figures to millions.

Cash was scarce, limiting project-specific work. Except for routine capital expenses and large-scale initiatives already in process, it was *slim pickings*. For this first postreorganization year, the amount for this work equated to less than $100/patient, company-wide, or slightly under $5 million.

For 700+ nursing homes.

I remember hearing a colleague say, "Don't spend it all in one place." We didn't, but were aggressive. On equipment. Mattresses. *Really good ones.*

Putting the company's money where our mouths were helped to legitimize what we were asking people to do. Our priorities? Developing leadership. Building nursing staff competence. Strengthening relationships with rehabilitation partners. Fortifying a commitment to patient care and quality assurance. In the process, using best approaches possible in coaching—defining what people were paid to do and what successful work performance looked like—we believed that investing in *superior* equipment would help hardworking people achieve and advance these priorities.

Upgrading mattresses, at least to some degree, was the goal for every company nursing home. This didn't require replacing every mattress. Some homes were on a replacement schedule, and others had used capital funding for this in prior years.

Defining the scope of work required field-based nursing consultants to conduct a full mattress inventory—home-by-home—by stripping beds and assessing mattress integrity during visits to individual homes.

This was hard and important work. Many sick patients defined *home* as their bed and mattress.

Priority status was assigned to the fifty homes with worst-in-class pressure injury performance. Halting and reversing results included eliminating equipment deficits as a scapegoat for piss-poor performance.

During inventory, company-wide leadership from Nursing, Rehabilitation Services, and Purchasing was invited to a "Bed Fair," where vendors displayed various beds and mattresses for evaluation and consideration.

This all-day event gave subject-matter experts time needed to share thoughts, ask questions, learn the features and benefits of items, and pick winners. This *Fair* was the first of many for the company and was repeated when considering equipment upgrades or other large-scale changes.

The inventory numbers were staggering. Nearly 20,000 mattresses were required to achieve full mattress integrity.

Even with immense corporate purchasing power, this initiative cost $6 million. Cash and capital limitations aside, it was a multiyear project.

These undertakings aren't like changing out your bedroom's Sealy Posturepedic. Retiring and installing new mattresses in a single nursing home is a team effort. Receiving and safely storing new ones—beyond a few—requires planning.

It's unsafe—and unwise—to stack new mattress boxes in a hallway, leaving them there until nursing, housekeeping, and maintenance workers are available to install. Left overnight in a nursing home's hallway, these new mattresses can become *unclaimed freight*, sold out of a box truck the following day.

Removing old inventory is a beast. Mattresses aren't resold on eBay or thrown in a dumpster. When left outside, they're a motel for critters you'd rather see in the woods. When done correctly, executing a wholesale mattress change takes several people and days.

ᔕ

We embarked on a three-year program, spending $2 million annually. Forty percent of the company's special project funding for Year One would be devoted to one line item, without true daylight on available funding in future years.

This project—and scale—was *very unpopular* among some company leaders. In saying YES to mattresses, something had to give, like delaying or reducing upgrades and renovations to some nursing homes, and responding "no" or "next year" to other well-designed and intended requests.

Leaders objected that this project conflicted with company norms and was contrary to their value structure.

By design, this project didn't differentiate by patient or payor. These upgrades—mattresses designed to provide pressure relief and additional comfort to patients—would be made available to all patients, including Medicaid patients.

Yes ... Medicaid patients. We thought: *Why not?*

Medicaid patients comprised the greatest number of patients served, and were the longest staying. As their nursing home stays lengthened, risks of skin breakdown escalated.

Additionally, our research indicated that the incidence rate of acquired pressure injuries was highest among Medicaid patients.

Critics viewed this approach as madness. To them, project-specific capital was essential to attract more premium paying Medicare and Managed Care admissions. Doing otherwise was *industrial blasphemy*.

Countering these sentiments, we shared that the universal indicator the public equated with nursing home quality—acquired pressure injuries—was nowhere near a source of company pride. Until then, establishing confidence among stakeholders was unattainable.

Soon after, critics softened. And the company's value structure shifted.

Concluding Year One, the company reduced its rate of acquired pressure injuries by half—from 8 percent to 4 percent. This was only the beginning.

Improvement continued over the succeeding four years. Concluding Year Five, this company-wide metric was a shade below 2 percent.

Mattress integrity alone wasn't this improvement's silver bullet. It did, however, hugely contribute in an incredibly large-scale approach to addressing skilled nursing's biggest embarrassment.

This project underscored the company's commitment to its patients, and to its workers. In this instance, the right equipment was available for workers to treat and serve patients, without the need for overcompensation for deficient or malfunctioning equipment.

Those other items ... surveys—*I mean, open book tests*, CMPs, per-for-mance? Over the five-year stretch, they improved too.

Without stepping over dollars to save pennies.

Good Grades Are Good Business

Wrapping up this chapter, one topic worth expanding upon is *passing the open book test* as a business strategy.

A search firm once approached me for a senior executive position with a publicly held nursing home company. Having competed against them for years, I had almost no knowledge about their people, approaches, and values.

The interview rotation included one-to-one time with the company's CEO. While he wouldn't be my boss, he would influence the hiring decision.

He asked how—during employment with *two* competing nursing home companies, in distinctly different markets—nursing homes I oversaw consistently outperformed those in his company, across multiple key performance indicators. His company was larger, older, and better resourced. Being outperformed didn't make sense.

I explained that every nursing home's business strategy contemplated a long-range time frame and sequential improvement—quarter-over-quarter and year-over-year.

At its foundation, the strategy included avoiding *any* business interruption.

Reflecting on my nursing home administrator experiences, I recounted the pain endured through such interruptions. Blowing a survey or needing to manage the aftermath of a verified complaint, driven by a handful of upset family members, seriously derailed a nursing home's momentum.

Continuing, I described a finite market supply of patients and workers, a low tolerance among medical and referral communities, and a nursing home's fragile goodwill. Lost business momentum and trust was never immediately regained. Every nursing home "was only as good as their last hit."

Like many winning teams, playing superior defense and capitalizing on the mistakes of competing nursing homes routinely resulted in market share gains. This occurred by taking very good care of patients and passing the open book test.

When our nursing homes remained in survey compliance and did not experience *any* business interruptions, we would expect the following to occur:

- The public and medical community would continue viewing us favorably.
- New referral activity would remain uninterrupted.
- Working environments would remain free of drama and knee-jerk decisions.
- Money would be used creatively, to "build a moat" between competitors.

While working to achieving this state, we'd wait—for as long as necessary. A competitor would eventually commit preparation and execution errors, experiencing their own case of "business interruptus."

This CEO was noticeably quiet throughout most of this exchange, responding with one follow-up question … "Can you do the same thing here?"

Not knowing the company's people, approaches, and values now placed me at a severe disadvantage. Plus, the nursing homes I'd overseen had been kicking the asses of his homes for more than ten years.

Thinking about it, I explained that executing this business strategy could be done with any nursing home, or nursing home company. This, however, required:

- **Patience.** It would not occur quickly.
- **Desire to change.** Old habits die hard.
- **Commitment.** Not everyone would want to do it.

Since this is a chapter on the open book test, I'll stay focused, sharing that this business strategy remains a winner, though every threat to success remains a reality.

Oh, the job … I got it and loved it. Over the next eight years, I saw this business strategy successfully executed—repeatedly.

WHAT YOU CAN DO

Ask Questions About:

- Surveys and simulated surveys. What are the historical results?
- Survey preparation techniques. What does the nursing home (or company do)? Are they unique? Are they effective?
- How is money spent to improve patient care?
- Equity among patients. Is investment based on payor re: beds, mattresses, therapy services?

- Pressure injury prevention and treatment. What does the home do, and how do they do it? What is (and isn't) working?

Look for...Everything! While Doing Your Own "Rounding":

- Visit places people rarely go. Tour the kitchen, laundry, and shower areas. What do you notice?
- Examine equipment condition and operability. Are items broken or out of service?

Listen to What People Say:

- Do caregivers talk being shorthanded, in anything?
- Do workers and leaders compare their home to competitors? What do they say?

VI

IMPORTANT PEOPLE DON'T TALK AND OTHERS DON'T LISTEN

An earlier chapter touched on the communication challenges physicians experience about death and dying. Understandably so. These are massively unpleasant topics. Generally, I've witnessed this when matters involving conflict, questions, or emotion exceed their comfort zones.

These important practitioners have admitted discomfort talking about hard things. Some avoid them entirely. Few take the awkward steps toward improving. Given the choice to talk about something hard—they'd rather not.

Stranded in this *desert of silence* are patients, families, and caregivers.

Being a physician is tough. Massive workloads, responsibilities, and expectations. Politics galore. Administrators and practice managers. Expecting physicians to become more like social workers is naive and misguided. When finding one skilled in communicating with clarity and ease, enjoy the benefit and good fortune.

Today, being seen *and* heard—is challenging. This isn't a secret.

There are, however, times when people don't want things seen and heard. Parts of personal and family histories. Embarrassing facts. Yet when these things aren't seen—or heard—they can risk what we treasure.

Why Talking Matters

As we age, we wrestle with secrets. Pride and ego can harm a nursing home patient. In their quality of life and care received, and in their longevity.

You see, patient records are one-dimensional. Even with superior charting and reporting, knowledge gaps about patient needs remain, making responses and behaviors unpredictable. Unpredictability creates surprises.

Patient interviews provide additional dimensions. Person-to-person conversations unearth facts and patterns, likes and dislikes, and short- and long-term histories, strengthening goals and approaches to providing best possible care.

Unfortunately, patients struggle with their stories. Sometimes, they're simply unable to share. Others resist, potentially adversely impacting the time, place, person, and approach to services received.

It's worth sharing that patients—and families too—aren't *graded* on their stories. Whatever it is, it's earned. A lifetime's résumé. While sometimes painful, these stories need sharing to equate the care and attention provided with a patient's life résumé.

Here's an example.

A person is admitted with a history of dementia, recently managed unsuccessfully at home. In her eighties, her history includes two marriages, each involving physically and verbally abusive husbands, producing bruises, broken bones, and other trauma.

In years preceding admission, she "swore off" men, becoming circumspect of all men in her life—including sons-in-law and physicians. Now, she's being placed in a memory care unit, among male patients and caregivers.

Upon admission, and days thereafter, this backstory hadn't been shared. People with the ability to share didn't, believing it was *no one's business*—until the patient initiated a physical altercation with a man seated beside her at mealtime, or a male caregiver triggered incredibly unpleasant memories.

Another more private and personal example involves continence—or the lack thereof. Some patients aren't hospitalized prior to admission, making it hard to assess their bowel or bladder condition and habits—especially when *they won't tell you.*

People sometimes overmanage this condition, risking terrible consequences. Incontinence episodes and walking to the bathroom unassisted have resulted in patients falling, and never getting up.

Histories of falling are untold secrets. Why? Walkers are for *old* people. Wheelchairs too. People fear being tied into bed. Family members resist disclosing a patient's falls history for fear of judgment that they didn't—or couldn't—prevent these falls.

Adding these important dimensions to their loved one's story make it easier for the nursing home to provide the best care possible—at the earliest opportunity.

They will provide a more complete picture for caregivers and decision-makers.

They always do.

Being Seen and Heard

Life changes for people responsible for nursing home patients. Communicating with the nursing home becomes a new feature of their lifestyle *for as long as it takes.*

This change adds much more to one's plate. Calls about changes in condition or medications. Falls and skin tears. Newfound requests for time, requiring attention, participation, decisions, and more.

Predictably, something *has* to give. Time-sensitive responsibilities—mail, bills, appointments, voicemails—might be deferred or ignored. Work, kids, partners, spouses, and friends can become diminished priorities.

And sometimes, their loved one—now safely admitted to the nursing home—can be forgotten, seen less, or rarely heard.

Serious family members and patient representatives, however, *never* miss a loved one's Patient Care Plan Conference.

Why? Attending, hearing, and sharing important information, and taking good notes at this conference gives a home the *best* opportunity to provide the *best* possible care and quality of life to their loved one.

Why? Time moves quickly. Patient experiences are dynamic. Missing a conference—or not participating fully—means delayed opportunities. You can gather and share information ahead of time so the best choices are made for care and everyone is working together.

When care conferences are missed, questions end up taking time away from the doctor–patient relationship.

If you catch an edge in my tone, it's because those responsible *frequently miss* patient care plan conferences.

Then we hear a lot of: "I didn't know."

Having been on both sides of this conversation—as administrator and family member—there are three-word responses to "I didn't know," like:

- "You weren't here."
- "You weren't listening."
- "You didn't care."

I ate these words as an administrator. Each was an invitation for family members to dial 1-800-I-HATE-THIS-NURSING-HOME, file a complaint, and outcome aside, ruin your day.

There are alternatives for the busy, whose calendars are double-parked. Meetings are available in person, by phone, or virtually. When schedules conflict, ask the nursing home to adjust, or select a designate. Then, reasons for suggested goals and approaches become known and understood, and you'll be able to fully support the person being cared for.

Clamming Up

Occasionally, important people create danger by intentionally suppressing critical information. Reasons vary by person and situation, with motivations and incentives behind this behavior beyond the scope of this chapter. Nevertheless, it happens. And people get hurt.

This instance involves an assisted living facility, rather than nursing home, though its features equally apply. I later was brought in as an expert witness for the defense of the assisted living facility in court. While I was not physically present for these events, I saw every bit of this patient's experience, afterward, via video.

A patient was hospitalized due to a fall that occurred at home.

During hospitalization, her family-provided medical history highlighted memory deficits. Her social history described support from outside services and frequent family member visits.

Prior to hospital discharge, the patient's daughter met with a sales representative for the assisted living provider, who conducted an on-site evaluation and completed an intake questionnaire. The patient was admitted to the assisted living facility the following day.

Nonemergency transporters brought the patient into the facility by wheelchair, secured at the waist with a seatbelt. While unextraordinary, this couldn't remain the standard for care at this location. Any device restricting freedom of movement would have been deemed a physical restraint, and incompatible with this care level and facility type.

Moments after seatbelt removal, the patient tumbled from the wheelchair to the floor. Being returned to the wheelchair by caregivers, this repeated—multiple times, with near identical outcomes, occurring within minutes.

Exhausting attempts to achieve safety while seated, caregivers secured a gait belt around the person's waist, testing her ability to walk with assistance. This proved fruitless, with multiple falls, pain and injury with each fall, and increased agitation with each interaction involving unfamiliar people.

Nearing the conclusion of this patient's one-day stay, three caregivers surrounded her—while seated or standing—as a rescue squad to prevent further pain, injury, and agitation. In serving this patient, each was diverted from providing care to others.

Over a few hours, this person fell, or was lowered to the floor, *nineteen* times.

Medical transportation workers returned, placed the patient on a gurney, and exited just a few hours after she had arrived.

This culminated in some severely upset people, including representatives of the discharging hospital and the rehospitalized patient's family. Eventually, the family sued the assisted living provider. Administrative action was taken against the facility's director of nursing, resulting in suspension of her nursing license.

Inarguably, serious mistakes were made during the on-site and intake performed by the assisted living facility's salesperson. Something incredibly important was missed. This person was never a candidate for this setting and would even be a challenge for most nursing homes.

Months after the suit's filing and administrative actions taken by the state's Board of Nursing, several items surfaced, including testimony that the intake performed was at surface depth, lacking the due diligence to determine placement suitability, and matching patient needs with the facility's competence and capacity.

Additionally, hospital caregivers testified that similar patterns of falling occurred during hospitalization, with the patient restrained in bed across her chest, waist, and legs—and bedcovers pulled up to her neck—during the on-site and intake visit.

Not a good look for the hospital, incentivized to find placement for *every* patient, nor the family member answering questions and providing medical history on behalf of the patient. Important people mishandled important information about this patient or made efforts to hide it.

The two-day hearing about the Board of Nursing sanctions ended quickly. Hospital caregivers' testimony found daylight, embarrassing those behind this action. Shortly thereafter, plaintiffs withdrew the civil action against the facility.

By then, extensive damage had been done. A patient had been terrorized, caregivers traumatized, and a nursing leader had been victimized.

This is what can happen when important people keep secrets or clam up.

Listen to Those Trusted Most

Nursing homes are busy places. Food, laundry, housekeeping, and medication carts driven throughout hallways. Patients in wheelchairs traveling to and from meals, activities, and showers.

Same is true in the therapy gym, or rehabilitation department. Physical, occupational, and speech therapy teams work on improving a patient's physical, functional, psychological, and cognitive condition.

When work centers around the patient, big things happen. They get stronger, living longer and happier lives, many times leaving the nursing home and returning home because the energy supplied by all parties—including the patient—is aligned.

When it isn't, achieving these outcomes is harder.

Important people, such as directors of nursing and teams, know this and share this with those they direct, displaying a partnership with rehabilitation leadership which permeates the home.

Leaders and caregivers mirror this behavior when interacting with the home's medical staff. Attending physicians vary widely, depending on the nursing home's size, physician specialty, and patients' conditions. Patient caseloads range from one to two per physician to half (or more) of a home's patient population.

Physicians working at nursing homes are doing the homes a huge favor. They're underpaid for their service; none of them are saying:

"I can't wait to work in a nursing home!"

Customer service can't be taken for granted. Busy as anyone, and difficult to replace, physician routines differ by:

- Visit schedules – early morning, midday, early evening
- Staff accompaniment – with nursing leadership or persons responsible for direct care
- Computer access – at the nursing station or in a private area
- Examination space – in a patient room or a distinct space

Their input helps optimize performance. When pursued and acted upon, patient care excellence is within reach. Otherwise, disenchantment builds. When it persists, physicians lose interest, hurting a home, its patients, and caregivers.

Directors of nursing and their leaders are tone-setters for physician work flow. These principles were introduced during their education, reinforced during clinical rotations, and demanded by superiors along their respective career paths.

Respecting the customer service skills that administrators bring to nursing homes, this element is routinely deferred to their nursing partners. Candidly, I did this while working as an administrator.

Why? When physicians are involved, nurses are superior in managing most anything.

Why? Because physicians trust nurses. So do Americans.

In *Gallup's* "2025 Honesty and Ethics Professions Rankings," nurses were first among all categories, with physicians a distant fourth.[86]

This has been the case for more than twenty consecutive years.

When trust is optimized, physicians optimize time with the patient. The home's reputation strengthens within the medical community, and help requests receive quick, drama-free attention.

Astute nurses know when to request a physician's help, and their patients reap the benefits. Their motto: Go early, and if necessary … go often.

Situations arise, however, where nurses and leaders don't speak up and let physicians know what's going on, hanging onto a problem too long, with the root cause a hypersensitivity to "bothering" someone—be it a supervisor or specialist.

When nurses are at loggerheads with families rejecting or refusing to accept a patient's planned goals, approaches, diets, or medications, this is incredibly unproductive, eroding trust in the nursing home, its caregivers, and its leadership.

The nursing home doesn't prevail in these arguments. Eroded family trust leads to complaints or negative word-of-mouth in the community.

During these arguments, patients routinely remain silent, avoiding their loved one's ire. Talk about important people *not* talking!

Before these flashpoints, however, the best nursing leaders seek counsel from attending physicians—or medical directors—to engage in managing or preventing this strife.

Trust—in Action

Nurses possess one final attribute solidifying their standing as the most trusted professionals: They usually know exactly what needs to be done. Deeply experienced in patient-centered care, resource allocation, teamwork, and business principles, nurses know how to get sh*t done.

Even before electronic records and AI, nurses solved problems, relying only on their heads, hearts, and hands, helping people live to see another day.

These attributes aren't distinct to nursing leaders. It's displayed departmentally—like a game of follow the leader—at patient admission, condition changes, physician interactions, and following diagnostic testing or hospitalization.

Its pervasiveness is unmistakable. This example highlights important people working together, for every nursing home patient. Its foundation is mathematically driven, using time, volume, and energy, measuring medication necessary to maintaining or improving their *overall* condition.

Here, the term *overall* includes the patient's physical, functional, psychological, and cognitive condition.

This isn't an independent study. Pharmacists conduct drug regimen reviews *monthly*, identifying irregularities in medications prescribed for *every single patient.*

This review sorts a patient's lineup card of drugs, looking for conflicts with diagnoses, adverse interactions with other drugs or known allergies, and dosage or duration anomalies, for starters.

Plus, prescribed and over-the-counter medications, over-the-counter items, and nutrition provided intravenously, including the method by which these items are administered.

For every single patient. Every single month.

Once completed, review findings are reported to the patient's attending physician, the director of nursing, and the home's medical director.

As an administrator, these reviews were a big deal. Before the digital age, reviews and responses were performed manually.

During reviews, nurses shared findings with attending physicians.

At conclusion—the consultant's exit conference—*we didn't go home.* The director of nursing, other nurses, and I remained until contacting each attending physician, sharing *every* patient-specific recommendation, and adding, adjusting, refining, discontinuing, and confirming each medication change.

Overkill? No way.

Personalize this. If told that among the medications, vitamins, and supplements you took, one or two were degrading your overall health, how long would you wait?

Between consultant visits, nurses put higher learning in play, sharing information on adverse drug-to-drug, drug-to-allergy, drug-to-diet, and drug-to-disease (or diagnosis) through the home's quality assurance efforts. This approach helped stave off many repeat occurrences and patient risks.

Subsequent reviews perpetuated this drill. Our goals:

- A shorter consultant report

- Fewer issues and changes
- Trending information for the home and each of its units

When we excelled, report recommendations were narrowed to the most recently admitted patients, further narrowing in succeeding months. Recommendations for longer-staying patients were limited, as nurses learned and knew more about their patients, addressing previously made recommendations.

These behaviors and results are common where talented, aligned leadership and a sense of urgency merge. Patients receive the best possible care, constantly involving physicians and *creating* time for other duties within nursing departments.

Additionally, rehabilitation departments operate on schedule. Patients keep appointments as absences due to adverse effects of drug-to-drug interactions and other complications subside.

This is what can happen when important people talk and listen—and continue doing so.

ೞ

As experienced, this *element* of the patient care model—medication management—is the most impactful to a home's ability to do *the right thing, in the right places, at the right time, to the right people, and for the right price.*

I'll share a story to illustrate.

I once asked a chief nursing officer to estimate the time required to properly prepare, deliver, and document administration of a patient's medication—making certain the *right* individual received the *right* medication, with the *right* dosage, at the *right* time, via the *right* route, with the *right* documentation and the *right* patient response.

Seven (7) *rights* defined success. Anything less could *kill a patient.*

This experienced and talented nurse responded: *three (3) minutes*. Though opinions may vary, this is the value used for *time*.

In a nursing home with 100 patients receiving care daily, and three minutes required to correctly administer medications to each, the incremental impact of two medications administered per patient equaled *ten (10) hours of nursing time daily.*

Surprised? Many industry veterans have been when this detail was provided:

Change in Meds/ Day/Patient		Minutes to Administer/Med	Time/Patient
2 medications/ patient/day	x	***3*** minutes/patient/medication	= ***6*** minutes/day

Time/Patient		# of Patients in a Nursing Home	Time/Day (minutes)
6 minutes/day	x	***100*** patients	= ***600*** minutes/day

Time/Day (minutes)		Minutes/Hour	Time/Day (hours)
600 minutes/day	÷	***60*** minutes/hour	= ***10*** hours/day

Here's what this means. From various sources, an average nursing home patient will take between 7–8 prescription and another 5 over-the-counter medications daily.

When the average number of medications administered per patient *increases by 2*, 10 hours of nursing time, daily, are required to satisfy this incremental work.

Conversely, when the average number of medications is *reduced by 2*, the amount of time saved is equal to ten hours.

This is nursing home math.

In the former case, additional worker hours may be required to satisfy this increase. Absent an increase, something important—which should be done—becomes secondary, or unimportant.

In the latter case, newly found time is available to address undone work, spend additional time with patients or one-to-one time with workers, or reduce the punishing effects of overtime.

Astute nurses know all of this, are serious about optimizing medications and working on reductions at every opportunity. Occasionally, they are strident and unyielding. Sometimes, they are complete assholes about it.

Good for them. They should be. As should the home's administrator.

Alternatively, nursing homes led by those not talking or listening enough, who don't get this dimension *right*, risk eventually getting almost everything else *wrong*.

In a few weeks, a month, or a quarter, the home's patient care indicators begin flashing *wrong*. But as the saying goes ... Wait for it.

Remember, a nursing home's patient flow is dynamic. Month-over-month, a home cares for different people, who are sicker at entry compared to those departing. Numerous medications are prescribed for hospitalized patients, with orders frequently landing on the patient's transfer sheet which accompanies them to the home.

Reflexively, nurses and attending physicians opt for continuity from one care setting to another, retaining hospital medication orders. When multiple patients are admitted on a day or shift—maybe, Fridays between 4:00 and 7:00 p.m.—this practice of copying over prior medication orders can become *automatic*.

Time is not anyone's friend. Orders need confirmation, charts need to be created and updated, and medications need to be ordered.

As patient stays lengthen, risk-creating dynamics compound. Multiple specialists overseeing care—geriatricians, psychiatrists, cardiologists, oncologists, neurologists, endocrinologists, podiatrists, dentists, pain management experts—each have views to what is *best* for patients, often without *complete* information of their histories or conditions.

Momentum develops in homes led by those not talking or listening enough. Pharmacy consultant visits occur with the director of nursing or administrator (or both) absent at exit. Electronically-produced recommendations will spend days or weeks in these leaders' inboxes, without review, distribution—*or action.*

Meanwhile, additional specialist visits, with medication orders prescribed by physicians lacking consultant recommendations, ensue.

Thanks for being patient while you ... *Waited for it.*

Embarrassingly, I've seen this happen. At, and above, an individual nursing home.

Root causes for this behavior pattern: a) *This is hard,* or b) *I don't want to do it.*

It is hard. This example illustrates how hard it can be. We'll take a step back in time and follow a patient.

A person experiences an event at home, resulting in hospitalization. They're scared, likely disoriented, possibly dehydrated and malnourished. They may be suffering from dementia.

While hospitalized, the patient displays behaviors consistent with fear, disorientation, dehydration, or malnutrition, and prescribed an antipsychotic to manage behaviors. These orders remain in place for the hospitalization's duration.

Upon nursing home admission, the patient's hospital medication orders are transferred, including the antipsychotic, and maintained in the nursing home's medication regimen.

Now, the *work is harder*. The risks become very high.

Determining this medication's continuation requires deep digging. Short-stay patients with antipsychotic medications are massive red flags for homes, indicating the need for mental health services that may or may not be immediately available or effective, *or* an inaccurate diagnosis that will require other skilled practitioners to resolve.

Risks heighten if this patient has dementia. Continuing antipsychotics usage likely increases the patient's mortality risk, as indicated by the

US Food and Drug Administration's (FDA) Black-Box warning issued regarding first- and second-generation antipsychotics (FGA/SGA).[87]

Alternatively, *not wanting to do it*—the convergence of leadership apathy, patient flow dynamics, and multiple practitioners—creates *medication mismanagement.*

Under these conditions, a patient can end up with twenty *or more* prescribed medications. At extremes, I've seen patients whose orders are double.

Imagine having orders for twenty-plus medications administered daily, requiring that each be taken *with water*. A robust appetite for food is gone, resulting from the water required to wash all this down or the side effects of this medication "salad." Sounds awful.

I won't criticize physicians for this development. They're working with the best information available at the time or as provided by others.

They'll tell you that with time and collaboration, they'll get it increasingly right. Because they don't always have the time or the opportunity to collaborate, they rely on the home's nursing department for help.

Help—defined as important people talking and listening. Why?

Physicians trust nurses and want to help in getting this dimension *right,* before almost everything else becomes *wrong.*

Getting it right is incredibly hard. It ...

- Requires daily effort
- Involves getting hands dirty in the details
- Demands disciplined, rigorous work to best serve patients and workers
- Needs important people talking—and listening

Communicating and Managing Expectations

This chapter of important people and their communication quality becomes complete by including bosses and direct reports, or workers and caregivers.

When first addressing colleagues—as administrator, middle manager, regional vice president, or company executive—I've said: "I'm going to ask you for the impossible, and then a little bit more."

Once hearing this, many faces went blank. If expressions spoke, they might've said ...

What's he mean by 'impossible'?

This guy is effed up.

I want to go home.

Coaching—through talking and listening—translated the impossible to achievable. Later, these colleagues coached others, pursuing and achieving incredibly lofty goals.

This work was fun. But it was *more fun to watch*.

In nursing homes, best coaching establishes clarity and agreement in:

- What work the person is paid to do
- How successful work performance is defined
- What needs to occur for the person to advance, in both pay and responsibility

This might seem easy. It isn't.

Broken Tools and Empty Toolboxes

Many nursing homes evaluate individual performance using a manual or AI-generated checklist of ten-to-twenty elements, completed, signed, and shared with workers. Once a year. *Maybe.*

This could summarize a home's approach to coaching.

Not much talking and listening required here. The work is completing the checklist. Checked box, a sigh of relief, and *fuhgeddaboudit* until next year.

Or worse.

Upon joining four different companies, employee satisfaction surveys of all workers—totaling thousands—included this unanimous response: "I have never received a performance evaluation." Yes. Illuminating.

Historically, industry veterans routinely spoke of receiving their last performance evaluation at a parent–teacher conference *as a high school student.*

My first, nonchecklist style, occurred fifteen years after my first day working in a home. This experience didn't endure. During my final twenty years in the business, I either received no performance evaluation, or *had to write it myself.*

Having coached numerous workers, athletes, and executives, the most worthwhile investment—in a person's success—is the time and attention to evaluating and coaching their performance.

Evaluating people can have a material impact on a nursing home. It requires a good faith attempt to assessing individual work quantity and quality, reinforcing desired outcomes and the preparation required to advance, in pay and responsibility.

Others concur with this viewpoint.

In the March-April 2019 *International Journal of Education and Science Research Review* article, "A Study on the Impact of Performance Appraisal Systems on Employee Motivation and Career Progression," researchers concluded that:

"Staff members report more work satisfaction, engagement, and loyalty to their organizations after participating in evaluation processes that are open, fair, and focused on professional growth."[88]

Investing in this environment won't guarantee every worker will achieve success. It will, however, guarantee each receives coaching—the opportunity to talk and listen. How workers apply coaching ultimately determines their degree of success.

ɞ

Again, this seems easy. Why doesn't it happen?

Here are some reasons, encompassing *all* business types:

- Companies don't know how to do evaluations.

- Companies don't know how to do them without making incredibly big mistakes.
- Companies don't find value in the cost of doing them.
- Companies would have to know what their employees are doing.

Companies committed to evaluating performance require *evaluators* to possess a variety of skills, including:

- Reading
- Writing
- Thinking
- Watching
- Listening
- Communicating
- Making decisions
- Delivering good and bad news
- Managing upset people
- Patience

Most skills are found in the poster capturing Robert Fulghum's, "All I really need to know I learned in kindergarten."[89] Nevertheless, skill deficiencies and absences among bosses and supervisors contribute to companies avoiding evaluations.

Massive Opportunities

In forgoing evaluations, companies forfeit the benefits of people growing beyond present roles, and their resultant career destinations.

Their histories are abundant. People whose careers began at hourly pay rates of $2.65, $3.10, or $3.35, with fascinating adventures, like:

- Administrators, whose master-level professional careers began as receptionists or billing clerks, with journeys including college degrees (sometimes), licenses to practice, miserable first assignments rejected by others, and professional ups and downs
- Directors of nursing, starting as nursing assistants or certified medication technicians, proceeding through multiyear and multidegree experiences, testing their fortitude to advance academically and endure plenty before becoming a nurse executive
- Senior vice presidents, first employed as activities director or staff nurses, whose careers were marked with promotions, demotions, transfers, employer changes, relocation, sales, mergers, expansions, reorganizations, and bankruptcies

The common denominators in their stories?

An important person or two—maybe, several—invested in talking and listening, possessing these beliefs:

- People will learn, develop, and become incredibly good at their jobs.
- People will prepare for growth and advancement opportunities.
- People will take advantage of opportunities that materially change their lives.
- People will stay with the nursing home or company which provides them the time and attention to learn and develop.

Yet this process is as *rare* as seeing an ivory-billed woodpecker in an Arkansas forest.

It is, however, what workers are starved for.

ᔓ

Preparing and participating in a *thousand-plus* performance evaluations, I've seen workers respond to this attention, conversation, learning and development firsthand.

Once initiated, evaluators can aid rather than drive this experience. Environments built on talking, listening, and opportunity allow workers to pave their own career paths.

And they will.

Dissecting these experiences, people displayed these characteristics in preparing for growth and advancement:

- **Willingness as a student.** Workers committed to learning and development are lifelong learners, returning to the role of student again and again. Many embraced lifelong learning professionally—and personally.
- **Patience and vision.** Workers understood experts weren't *born*, and that most are novices when attempting something new. Additionally, the value of time—to attempt, fail, regroup, examine, and repeat—helped realize individual ambitions.

  Patience was routinely tested. Dormant skills and techniques often required renewal, especially for workers moving from subject-matter expert or line manager to consultant, *and* those whose small-scale subject-matter expertise was broadened to include supervising others at regionally, divisionally, or company-wide.

- **Discipline.** Simply stated, workers focused on their own improvement. With additional effort, improvement accelerated, nearing or achieving excellence.

  The relationship between discipline and baseline talent bears comment. Workers possessing less pure talent, yet applied more discipline to study and preparation, enjoyed better results than those banking on talent alone. However, remarkable growth was realized when talented workers added discipline to their learning and development.
- **Rigorous preparation and repetition.** In addition to company or industry-sponsored learning opportunities, workers converted their own private, personal time to practice time, with extra effort directed to building competence in new skills and techniques.
- **Manageable performance anxiety.** Return demonstration required learners to "show off" to peers and superiors, testing their fear and risk of failure, and gaining comfort with newly-developed skill sets.
- **Receptivity to advanced coaching.** Workers grew to accept more exacting feedback while learning and developing. This included a first introduction to superiors, or *managing up*, with progress in newly-built skills increasingly evaluated. Coaching changed in tone and tempo, preparing the worker for demanding future experiences.

Workers committed to their own learning and development were recognized for their efforts with applause and respect. But it's worth noting that all coaching experiences weren't celebratory. Others whose progress fell short or displayed a lack of effort in preparation risked bruised feelings or a good old-fashioned ass-chewing—which is yet another form of talking and listening.

Barrier-Driven Behaviors

Talking and listening isn't so easy anymore. Our world is different.

People no longer engage in discourse. Phones have become appendages, a substitute for the fidget spinner, or their best friend.

These changes are impactful. Communication deficits are crippling, especially in nursing homes, which depends on teamwork in a dynamic environment where errors, omissions, and shortcomings affect people.

My fear? This trend never reverses.

This section summarizes root causes that cripple talking and listening between important people—applicable across the spectrum of those intended to place patients or workers at each conversation's center.

Here are the first five:

- People can't write. And since they can't, they won't.
- People don't ask for input from others.
- People don't develop coaches.
- People are evolving into social misfits.
- People resist one-to-one conversations.

I once had a boss, who, before a brief conversation with me, said he'd speak from a prepared script, protecting against miscommunicating points he wanted to share with me.

Adding further color, he also shared that when speaking to his spouse and children about important familial matters, he preferred reading from a script—while seated at the family table—so that points made, or words chosen were not misinterpreted or criticized.

This is intimate communication in the digital age.

ꕥ

***Occam's razor*, a principle which eliminates extraneous assumptions,** resulting in the *simplest* answer being the *correct* one, helped determine the final root cause:

- People are satisfied being lazy.

Yes. This might be the simplest root cause for nursing homes underinvesting in talking and listening to workers. Why?

They don't want to do it. And no one can *make* them.

Often in life people are lazy. Nursing homes—and their companies—are no different. Plenty is chosen to *not* be done, usually involving voices from the top, accompanied by reasons this home or company—doesn't or shouldn't do it.

Leadership never states, "We don't do it here, because we just don't want to." Refreshing honesty is a rarity.

Instead, these statements become questions. Joining a company with no history of leadership development or performance evaluation, I shared plans to initiate each with the company's chairperson, who responded: "Are you serious?"

In another company, the underinvestment in workforce learning and development—purposeful performance management techniques, strategically building depth, planned retention approaches—was be summarized as: "Too corporate."

Yet, nursing homes and their companies make these choices. No one can *make* them do it differently.

Companies sometimes attempt threading the needle, purporting an investment in learning and development, while taking the laziest approach possible.

This example recounts a year-end performance evaluation with my boss.

This company's senior management team was made up of nearly twenty executives. Below illustrates the boss's organizational chart:

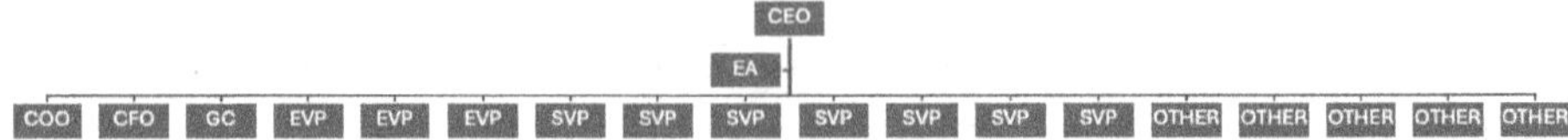

A span of control as wide as the Grand Canyon. This design required senior managers to learn and develop by accessing outside resources. The boss's time and attention was scarce. Talking and listening was something direct reports did among themselves.

My assignment? Complete my evaluation. Not a *self*-evaluation to match with the supervisor's, but the sole document used to evaluate my work, comparing performance to a series of measures.

Prior to submission to the boss, many senior execs shared their preliminary *self*-prepared evaluations with each other, to fact check and review for bias. Some were bold enough to share this work with trusted colleagues and direct reports.

Once finalized, my boss received a copy, in advance of the two-hour, one-to-one conversation.

Miserable … it was. Annually, for two hours, you learned—from your *self*-prepared evaluation—exactly where, how much, at what, and why you sucked at your job.

Debates during one-to-ones were lively, sometimes becoming personal. Understandably so. When your work no longer affected you personally, it was no longer worth doing.

Crying or tearing up during one-to-ones marked the beginning of an executive's end. Nevertheless, it did happen. Senior leaders were *reassigned* shortly thereafter, followed by internal job postings or calendar requests to participate in replacement interviews.

Eliminating someone over "water works" during the evaluation—that *they* wrote?

Lazy.

When Talking and Listening Worked

We'll end this chapter with a story where strategies and tactics shared earlier produced big victories for one nursing home.

I became this home's administrator after a company reorganization. The director of nursing was tenured and effective. Popular and beloved. Deservedly so. The workforce's core—intact for years—had an average age over fifty, with many related through birth or marriage, high school or nursing school classmates, or friends and work sisters. The balance of the crew was twentysomethings and recent high school graduates in first nursing home jobs, or searching for someplace worth landing—*and staying*.

Retaining veteran workers wasn't challenging. My nursing partner knew each of them, as she'd been evaluating performance of every caregiver for years. Retaining the less-tenured, however, was challenging. More time, attention, and direction would be required to maintain their interest, improve performance, and provide reasons for staying.

We needed coaches—people who supervised nurses and certified nursing assistants daily—to reach beyond technical expertise, explore advanced management techniques, and test their writing, listening, and relationship-building skills. Candidates initially resisted this idea, viewing it as "not nursing."

They were correct—sort of. These discrete topics aren't found in a class syllabus for anatomy, physiology, psychology, or pharmacology. Nevertheless, the home's ability to maintain and enhance its long-term ability to care for people—patients and caregivers—depended on their coaching ability.

Rather than using the *See One, Do One, Teach One* education approach, developing these nurses *as coaches* required an understanding of the "What" and "Why" behind *everything* before they were able to do *anything*. A poverty of time required building upon existing leadership muscle to satisfy their skepticism or anxieties. Within six months, this nursing home had several coaches equipped to evaluate nurses and certified nursing assistants (CNAs) and host one-to-one conversations.

Coaches ended up with spans of control ranging from eight to fifteen workers. The director of nursing and assistant director owned a slightly larger range compared to charge nurses, though several coaches requested expanded responsibilities.

To overcome growing pains, coaches paired up in one-to-ones. While one coach hosted a one-to-one conversation, the other watched and listened.

Coaching frequently exceeded reviewing what workers were paid for. Once establishing mutual trust, conversations commonly involved impactful issues frequently taken for granted, like relationships, parenting, domestic abuse, financial planning, and learning *how to perform* everyday tasks.

Coaches and workers were talking and listening. *They were also staying.*

ᔓᔕ

Upon joining this nursing home, Mondays meant new employee orientation. Newly-hired people spent classroom time with the home's staff development coordinator, then reported to their respective departments and supervisors for additional orientation.

During orientation, I'd spend thirty minutes with participants, introducing the company operating the home and its priorities, with Q&A to follow.

Eventually, my calendar no longer included Orientation Mondays. I found the staff development coordinator and applied my own version of the five *Whys (plus 1)*. It went like this:

Q: Why have we stopped doing Orientation Mondays?

A: *We don't need to do them weekly.*

Q: Why don't we have to do them weekly?

A: *We don't have new hires.*

Q: Why don't we have new hires?

A: *We don't need new hires. Part-timers are picking up more shifts. Some have become full-timers.*

Q: Why don't we need new hires?

A: *People aren't leaving.*

Q: Why aren't people leaving?

A: *People like it here.*

Q: Why do people like it here?

A: *Because people are paying attention to them.*

This nursing home went Orientation Monday-free for fourteen *months*.

Big things happened here. The nursing home was routinely within a patient or two of being fully occupied. Patient mix was routinely healthy, and we were paid timely, little going uncollected. *Translation:* The community was buying what we were selling.

Time saved from new-hire orientation activities allowed the home's staff development coordinator (a nurse practitioner) to help workers grow in areas beyond their core skills.

When people wanted to learn something new or different, time was available for this *highly competent, advanced practice registered nurse* to give people—individually or in small groups—the attention needed to build beyond the basics.

For example, many CNAs successfully completed the requirements to become a Certified Medication Technician (CMT). Multiple CMTs available on each day and shift meant nurses no longer had to "ride the cart," spending large chunks of a shift focused on passing routine medications. Additionally, CMTs advanced their own career development, gaining confidence through greater responsibility, and improving their pay.

Talking and listening, focused differently, also paid off in other ways.

The home's state survey resulted in one deficiency, and no complaint surveys. Patient restraints and acquired pressure injuries were at or near absolute *zero*. Few patients fell, and even fewer experienced unexpected weight loss. While there was much more to celebrate, I'll stop here.

Working at this home remains a career highlight. It was the last home where I served as an administrator.

Seventeen months after joining this home, I was promoted to territory manager. By the same company that had nearly sent me packing.

For years afterward, across several companies, developing coaches became central to business planning activities. In later, larger roles, I routinely recounted administrator experiences, encouraging leaders to build worker depth and skill, create learning environments promoting development, and giving people reasons to keep coming back—and consciously choosing to stay with their employer—through talking and, more importantly, actively listening.

WHAT YOU CAN DO

Ask Questions About:

- Patient care planning, and how it works—for you.
- Drug regimen reviews. The average medications per patient, and priorities for improvement.
- How people are coached and evaluated.
- Internal promotions and the stories behind people and their name tags.

Look for:

- Teamwork between nurses and physicians (or extenders, e.g., nurse practitioners)
- Leadership visible "on the floor."

Listen to What People Say:

- Focus on conversations between caregivers and their supervisors.

VII

AGENTS OF CHANGE ... AREN'T

In preparing this chapter, I reviewed books and reports from experts and thought leaders, seeking insights and opinions to enhance the reader experience, and facts about nursing homes that are not commonly known. I think this one fits.

Here goes, from the "Introduction and Summary" prepared by the Institute of Medicine's Committee on Nursing Home Regulation:

- A free market for nursing home care will remain a theoretical concept until a major portion of the financing of long-term care services has shifted from public sources (primarily Medicaid) to private insurance. *This is not likely to occur very soon.*
- Because of the cost, few individuals or families can afford a prolonged nursing home stay. As a result, Medicaid assists in paying for more than *60 percent* of all care. In most states, Medicaid rates are lower than those paid by private residents.
- The nursing home market is in fact two markets—a *preferential* one for those who can pay their way, and a second, more *restricted* one, for those whose stays are paid by Medicaid.
- Providers, consumer advocates, and government regulators *are all dissatisfied* with specific aspects of the regulations and the way they are administered.

- Providing consistently high quality care in nursing homes to a varied group of frail, very old residents, many of whom have mental impairments as well as physical disabilities, requires that the functional, medical, social, and psychological needs of residents be *individually determined* and met by careful assessment and care planning—steps that require professional skill and judgment. This process must be repeated periodically and the care plans adjusted appropriately.
- Not all nursing homes *have enough professional staff* who are trained and motivated to carry out tasks competently, consistently, and periodically.
- To hold down costs, most of the care is provided by nurse's aides who are *paid very little*, *receive relatively little training*, are *inadequately supervised*, and are *required to care for more residents than they can serve properly.*
- The turnover rate of nurse's aides is usually very high—from 70 percent to over 100 percent per year—a factor that *causes stress in resident-staff interactions*.[90]

These bulleted points may appear pedestrian. In this chapter's context, however, I believe they're material.

Why?

Because they were prepared not in 2025 or even 2020 but in … 1986.

Ronald Reagan was president and *Top Gun* debuted in theaters. It was the Decade of Decadence. Parachute pants. Big hair. Aqua Net hairspray was second to coffee.

This report, "Improving the Quality of Care in Nursing Homes," became required reading among industry professionals.

Nearly forty years later, Donald Trump is president, Netflix has taken the place of the local movie theater, AI is not BS, and Bitcoin is being talked about as an alternative to gold.

Incredible change over four decades. Except in the nursing home business.

Today, nursing home owners, executives and influencers, regulators, and lawmakers would likely find these points correct, or directionally accurate:

- A *major* portion of the financing of long-term care services continues to come from public sources (e.g., Medicare, Medicare Advantage, Medicaid).
- *Well over* half of nursing home revenues come from appropriated state and federal funding through Medicaid. As of July 2024, ***63 percent*** of US nursing home patients were receiving Medicaid coverage.[91]
- Due to cost, *few* individuals or families can afford a prolonged nursing home stay. In most states, Medicaid rates continue to be lower than those paid by private residents.
- The nursing home market consists of multiple tiers (and tiers within tiers) reliant *almost exclusively* on taxpayer-funded payors.
- Providers, consumer advocates, and government regulators *continue* to decry the administration of survey and enforcement of state and federal regulations.
- Nursing homes *remain challenged* in having enough professional staff trained and motivated to carry out these tasks competently, consistently, and periodically.
- CNAs *continue to provide* the bulk of direct care in many nursing homes, are paid very little, receive relatively little training, are at risk of being inadequately supervised, and can be required to care for more residents than they can serve properly.

- The turnover rate of nurse's aides *remains very high*—from 70 percent to over 100 percent per year (or more) and remains a factor that causes stress in resident-staff interactions.

Considering the massive change during the years 1986–2025, it's hard to imagine that the issues—or threats—which once plagued this industry remain.

This chapter touches upon forces presumed to be industrial change agents, yet by all accounts—over four decades—haven't.

The Newsroom

You may have heard of:

- St. Rita's Nursing Home (LA) and Hurricane Katrina
- The Rehabilitation Center at Hollywood Hills (FL) and Hurricane Irma
- Life Care Center of Kirkland (WA) and COVID-19

Regionally or nationally, these locations (or former locations) are well known, due to the media—whose mantra is, "If it bleeds, it leads ..."

In smaller markets, the ignominy of nursing homes is superseded only by events that drive more click-throughs or fit more coveted narratives of news outlets.

As a result, storytellers, or the risk of stories being told, are among the *hottest buttons* to senior executives and owners.

For many, hiding is preferred when the sh*t hits the proverbial fan. Anything that exposes names, faces, net worth, annual compensation, or known associates and their stories is better left buried.

Why? I'd be guessing. Doesn't make it less true.

When sharing unpleasantries, I've had superiors behave as if invaded by aliens, immediately uttering ...

"Whatever you do ... don't let the press find out!"

This mandate stifles full and timely disclosure, inviting explosive penalties and punishment to a home, a company, and its leadership.

In one company, receiving this demand after informing the company's chairperson of an elopement, I had to explain the communication processes to first-responder agencies and on-the-beat surveillance routinely conducted by the local press.

This exchange resulted in me receiving an old-fashioned tongue-lashing.

In another company, similar demands were issued by the company's CEO, after providing information about alleged sexual abuse of a patient. Receiving instructions to "stop the press," I proceeded to share—with him—the role of law enforcement investigating this allegation, the home's mandatory reporting requirements, and the substantial reach of the internet, social media, and its users.

This resulted in silence, later becoming a supernatural ass-kicking.

These interventions pale compared to seeing your name, in bold, jet black, Times New Roman, 36-font print, above the fold on page one of any newspaper's business section, or on page two of the local and national news section. These spots are reserved for people responsible for massively positive achievements, or being selected as ... asshole of the day.

During my career, I've been both, and still have the clippings.

Television also broadcasts misfortunes of the nation's nursing homes. Film crews entered nursing homes—most, uninvitedly so—where I was administrator or director of operations, looking for a live look-in based on calls from family members or anonymous sources, or requests for background, B-roll, or thirty seconds of Q&A regarding issues involving seniors, nursing homes, proposed legislation, or state lawmaker jousting matches with their governors over Medicaid funding.

This is life in the nursing home business. It's unavoidable.

One final story involves tragedy, a nursing home worker and law enforcement investigations captivating the local press and introducing a dimension familiar to readers, viewers, and listeners—fear.

When publicized, this incredibly unfortunate event—specifically, death—became an instant moneymaker. Papers were sold, unpaid media time grabbed, and political party leaders impressed.

One reporter picked up and ran with this story. The worker's death, by suicide, was front-page news, replaced later with personal diary excerpts, later followed with articles about the nursing home and company. The latter is unsurprising. Nursing home exploits neatly fit fear-based narratives. A home's Statement of Deficiencies is fertile ground for an enterprising reporter.

This reporting captured the interest of the local district attorney, and eventually the state's attorney general. Avoiding competition for ink space, they joined hands, dominating headlines and commentary, creating leverage at every opportunity. The words *criminal* and *civil* punctuated every sound bite.

Why? Because they could. And the newspaper *could ... not ... get ... enough ... of ... this.*

Storylines gained momentum. Fear did too. Everyday people, working at this nursing home, became scared.

- Scared to make a mistake
- Scared to talk to someone they didn't know
- Scared to have their name tag visible outside the workplace
- Scared to do their job as best they could

Some became so scared, they stopped coming to work all together.

As this unfolded, the company's VP of public relations arranged a meeting with the newspaper's editorial board.

The editors had prepared questions—covering facts and feelings, personal and business—taking notes throughout our conversation.

With litigation expected to follow, we set aside certain questions. This angered editors, responding that *their readers deserved to know.*

Completing their inquiries, they asked if I had any questions. I asked them a few:

- Had any of them ever worked in a nursing home? *They hadn't.*
- Did they know someone who had ever worked in a nursing home? *A few did.*
- Were the people they knew, who had worked in a home, good people? *They were.*
- Had they ever visited the nursing home about which they were writing? *They hadn't.*
- Did they really believe that people working in the nursing home were criminals? *Silence.*

Leaving this meeting, there's no way of knowing what transpired afterward. The nursing home and the company weren't out of the news for some time, though the tone tilted, somewhat.

Nevertheless, people remain scared. And this nursing home never bounced back from this experience.

After hours of programming from ABC's *Nightline* and *20/20*, CBS' *60 Minutes*, NBC's *Dateline*, and countless news sources—and the corresponding attention, rhetoric, facts and figures, expert insight, outrage, and shaming, these questions bear asking:

- Over nearly forty years, has the work of *the newsroom* made any difference?
- Or did they just sell papers, ad space and time, page views, and click-throughs?

Patient Care Litigation—History Worth Knowing

During the 1970s and 1980s, nursing homes were usually sued for instances of bad luck, strategy and decision-making, timing, or behavior. Legal challenges commonly involved state or federal enforcement actions resulting from survey performance, duration-of-stay contracting for private paying patients, or another anomaly.

Nursing homes were still in their industrial infancy. Though unthinkable today, for example, a patient care standard was physically restraining people to prevent falling.

Patients, with frailties and feelings, made for an unpredictable living environment. People fell, medication errors occurred, pressure sores developed. This happened then, and continues today.

ଓ

Employed as a territory and regional manager in the early nineties, most patient care events were managed locally and regionally.

After reporting events through the company's Operations and Nursing organizational hierarchy, risk management and legal leadership, service recovery efforts—including conversations with the patient and/or their representatives—routinely occurred with leaders closest to the home.

In these circumstances, I'd find myself partnered with a company representative, meeting with parties close to the patient who had experienced something unwelcome or unexpected.

Our guiding principles were:

- Hurting nursing home patients is not OK.
- When hurt, nursing home patients ought to have an approach available to remedy injuries.
- In the long run, this approach *ought* to change and improve nursing homes.

Conversations were unpleasant, and expectedly so. Eventually, this question was asked:

"What will it take to make this right for you?"

This placed control with the patient and their representatives. Many accepted this, articulating varying remedies:

- A meeting with workers involved or witnessing the event
- Reassignment or termination of specific workers
- Selection of specific workers for future care needs
- Compensation for medical bills
- Compensation for aggravation, pain and suffering, or a breach of trust
- Writing-off outstanding account balances for services previously provided
- Credits toward future charges incurred
- Transfer to another nursing home

Successful resolution depended on all parties being open-minded. Settlement authority varied by company, dependent on the event's nature and severity, and skills of company representatives.

While imperfect, this process worked. Pissed-off people defined and found satisfaction, without delay or deflection. Compensatory awards weren't carved up or diluted. Posturing was minimal. These were learning experiences, for the nursing home involved and territory, region, and company leaders.

When resolution couldn't be achieved locally, senior leadership would intervene. My senior leadership experiences included conversations with company risk management people, working to determine options and amounts for patients and their representatives to consider. These situations involved larger compensation amounts, and included features listed above that local leadership rejected in preliminary conversations.

Monetary amounts varied by situation. Determining suggested settlement amounts considered a patient's infirmity, age-based life expectancy prior to admission, income or earning capacity, and responsibilities associated with caring for, or raising, children under eighteen.

This wasn't breakthrough territory, and was intended to somewhat align with the existing award structures for personal injuries, recognizing elements pertinent to economic and noneconomic damages.

During this time, many states had limits (or caps) specific to personal injury cases—for punitive and noneconomic damages—influencing the number and type of cases filed for patient care events, and the amount of financial opportunity available to plaintiffs and the firms representing them.

ꕤ

By the mid-1990s, all this history ... *was history*.

States, with Florida and California serving as vanguard, changed the complexion for the nursing home industry. *Forever.*

Florida changed laws governing nursing homes and introduced a *patient's bill of rights*. In amendments, patients and their representatives could file civil suits for violation of their rights, with uncapped limits on compensatory and punitive damages, *and the inclusion of attorney's fees.*[92]

California's approach mirrored Florida's, using their Elder Abuse and Dependent Adult Civil Protection Act as the fulcrum for *attorneys to recover fees and related costs associated with litigation of a patient-related claim.*[93]

In future years, other states followed, introducing terms like *intentional harm, reckless or willful disregard, indifference to the rights of others, gross negligence, and malice.*

This legislative shift launched a new industry, involving lawyers, patients, nursing homes—and *lots* of money. *Lots.*

These legislative changes created new territory for lobbyists, paid to make their points known. Nursing homes, through their state and national trade associations, used lobbyists to counteract pro-plaintiff bar spokespersons, whose messaging favored newly-enacted laws, or amended old ones.

Reflexively and strategically, law firms added nursing home malpractice to their scope of services, renting billboards—sometimes right above a home—advertising this expanded, or newly-formed specialty.

ꕥ

Unless touched by sheer luck, every winner has a strategy. Contests involving the legal and nursing home professions relied on strategies frequently including these tactics:

- Sustaining or enhancing laws most favorable to *the cause*
- Exerting maximum leverage with *existing intelligence*
- Recognizing the premium effect of *fear*
- Converting fear into *hatred*
- Daring the weak to *defend themselves*

Lobbying strategies were simple—for the bar and the industry. Plaintiff firms desired a national landscape with laws favorable for compensatory and punitive damages. No caps, and full recognition of attorney fees. Nursing homes defined successful legislation by capping punitive damages and limiting attorney fees.

This full-scale tug-of-war involved many matches and hours spent educating legislators and legislative aides. I participated in many of these conversations, across the country, accompanying company-employed and independent lobbyists.

The implications of these challenges are historically significant. Nursing home companies have intentionally sold or closed individual homes, consolidated homes in the same market, or completely exited states where the laws were deemed so unfavorable that continuing operations threatened the company's continued existence.

I witnessed this while working for companies with nursing homes operating in Florida, California, Mississippi, and Arkansas. Decisions were made to "wave the white flag" and adjust to these environmental forces or allow another company—in this case, ones able to organize each nursing home with sufficient legal insulation—to protect these homes against potentially ruinous litigation.

Presuming that these legislative dynamics apply only to the nation's worst nursing homes would be incomplete. It's quite the contrary. Location and legislative landscape are the *sole* determinants of high-volume, high-stakes patient care litigation activity.

It's much like mining for gold. If the all-in *cost* of finding and extracting an ounce of gold in a certain location *is greater than the market price* per ounce, there's sensibility in waiting to mine that ounce until the economic conditions change.

Calculations among plaintiff firms are no different. If it's too expensive to generate an attractive return on work performed in a specific state, firms will migrate to states where the returns are more favorable. These states provide what is referred to as "target-rich environments."

It's noteworthy that in the extreme, regulation and patient care litigation have driven companies from the US, surrendering their domestic core business and retreating to markets deemed safer.

After a long history of patient care litigation and regulatory distress, one company made a literal run for the border. In 2014, Extendicare Health Services, Inc., following their $38 million settlement with the US Department of Justice (DOJ), and the US Department of Health and Human Services, Office of Inspector General, decided that they'd had enough. Touted by the DOJ as "the largest *failure of care* settlement with a chain-wide skilled nursing facility in the department's history"—encompassing nursing homes in eight states, with deficient practices noted in staffing, catheter care, pressure ulcers and falls—the company made plan to move to "The Great White North."[94]

Upon settling with the Feds for alleged transgressions spanning from 2007–2013, their corporate secretary—in a November 10, 2014, *McKnight's* article, "Extendicare to sell US businesses for $870 million"—commented: "The US is a very volatile and risky environment. Canada is more stable."[95]

By July 1, 2015, Extendicare closed its deal with private-equity heavyweight Formation Capital, began closing their US operations in Milwaukee, and never returned.[96]

Other People's Work

As patient care malpractice requires an individual, an event, and an undesirable outcome involving medical and patient care provided (or not), this hasn't been the preferred strategy in suing nursing homes.

Though something unwanted *might* have happened to the patient, there's great risk to a case tried which concentrates on the patient's health, history, comorbidities, cognition, and behavior, or the skills and techniques possessed by involved caregivers at the time of the event.

This would make the case solely about everyday people. And people—namely, juries—generally don't like hurting people, especially when it involves errors committed through honest effort.

Instead, cases hugely discount the "medicine," and spotlight the nursing home.

Why? Homes are much easier targets. And substantial work on the matter already exists—*free*. It's easy for plaintiff firms to use a nursing home's Statement of Deficiencies and Plan of Correction (CMS-2567)—created by state survey agencies—as a road map. This makes it hard for nursing home leadership and defense firms to *play offense*.

Even in situations where survey documents make no reference to *the* specific event or patient involved in a case, it helps plaintiff firms advance or validate approaches to indict the nursing home.

Translation: *If the state says the nursing home sucks ... it must. Since the home sucks, our claim must be just.*

In addition, plaintiff and defense counsel use information that was paid for by parties involved *in prior cases*. This information is frequently used to advance an argument or impeach a witness, depending on the side represented and the circumstances involved.

This reality came into sharp focus following an in-person deposition, taking place at the plaintiff firm's law offices. At the deposition's conclusion, the firm's founding partner, who I'd met and been deposed by previously, entered the room to say hello, offering a tour of the offices. While impressive, they possessed an area I'd not experienced before, in any law firm.

Turning a hallway corner, we entered a large records storage area, measuring at least 20' x 30', with industrial shelving reaching 8' high. Boxes of case files covered nearly every square inch of the shelves. The floor was spotless, the room was climate-controlled, and with a little work, surgery might have been able to be performed within.

Curiously, and without subtlety, I began to look at labels on case file boxes. Several had names of nursing homes of which I was familiar. Watching me, my attorney/tour guide said, "You should know many of these nursing homes. This whole room is dedicated to work involving your company."

As this nursing home company was several hundred homes in size, it was surprising on one hand, and not so much on the other. Nevertheless, it left a mark, evidenced by this recounting.

Our tour wasn't finished.

Before departing this area, he directed my attention to a bank of shelves lining one of the room's four walls, stacked with boxes from floor to ceiling. Viewing these units, he said: "See these? All these boxes are yours. We have everything you've ever said in here."

In a world before AI, this firm—and others like it—built data warehouses on companies and their executives, using press releases, investor presentations, audio and video footage from company and industry events, video and hard copies of depositions and courtroom testimony, and any other publicly available or "on the record" documents.

When they needed them, they used them.

What a way to make a person want to watch what they said and keep their stories straight.

"Secret Agent" Intelligence

Inquisitors want to know everything about you and your company. Predictably, plaintiff firms rely on former workers and *moles* for intelligence on nursing homes and companies during legal action.

Lengths to which this intelligence is sought can be boundless. Here's more ...

In the late 1990s, I had a big job with a large company, with public visibility. One Saturday morning, arriving at the building, a few cars were parked in its lot. People were in to catch up, or prep for the week ahead. Entering my office, I found the lights on, with two people inside.

One was the company's contracted private investigator. The other, a complete stranger. Their undivided attention focused on a small case that was tracing horizontal lines of red light from the point at which the office walls and ceiling met, spiraling downward across its interior perimeter, one after another, separated by fractions of inches.

Asked to find another place to work until their work was completed, I questioned what was going on. They said, "We're sweeping your office for bugs. When we're done, we have two more to sweep."

About an hour later, these agents found me in a nearby conference room, sharing two very small items, the likes that might have been found in cracking open an old transistor radio or a TI-35 calculator.

These were *bugs*. Listening devices. One was behind the seam in a wallpaper strip, near a conference table. A second was inside a lamp near my telephone, in a place where only people like these men would consider looking.

For years afterward, sweeps continued every few months. Occasionally, devices were found in phones and behind switch plates.

After a while, knowing that this level of interest (or surveillance) wasn't just possible—*but likely*—became the standard in my working day routine.

This isn't just unfair ... it is illegal. It's done every day by people who are paid to win.

Fear as an Asset

If the legislative process is a tug-of-war, litigation is a street fight. Everyone gets hit and bruised. Some suffer lacerations. Some tap out early on.

"Going the distance" means battling societal attitudes, specifically those involving *fear.*

Plaintiff lawyers take center stage, selling *fear* to those prone to embracing that nursing homes are the *scariest places not located on Elm Street.*

With refined and gentle sales techniques, they drape *fear* in this messaging:

- Bad things happen in scary places.
- Scary people work in scary places.
- You should be afraid of scary places.
- Nursing homes are scary places.
- Bad things happen in nursing homes.
- People working in nursing homes are scary people.
- *You should be afraid of nursing homes.*

In doing so, they scare the bejesus out of nursing home leaders, their lawyers, and insurance people.

Inside a courtroom, they scare the bejesus out of jury members too.

One fear-inducing courtroom technique uses images of patients—*in Technicolor*. Photographs, blown up bigger than a *Fathead*, are placed on an easel, showing a nursing home patient at a family wedding or birthday party, full of smiles. Beside it is one taken a day (or several) following a fall.

If you've seen an elderly parent or grandparent days after a bump or fall at home, you might have been shocked. I'll admit—my first time, experienced as a teenager—was a stunner.

Later, I learned the reasons why nursing home patients, who—after falling out of bed—could end up looking like they'd taken a knockout punch.

Thinning skin, medications, or vitamin deficiencies place nursing home patients at a greater risk of bruising.

As we age, this will probably happen to us too.

Nevertheless, a patient's discolored face, with shades of black, red, purple, green, yellow, and brown, on a poster four feet wide by six, seven, or eight feet high, leaves jurors with images which can't be unseen. Posters remain in plain view until sufficiently striking fear in jury members.

Displays aren't limited to patients' faces. Pressure injuries cases are treated similarly. Heels, elbows, or sacral areas are enhanced to sizes making the bodily features near unrecognizable, intending to induce nausea, tears, or terror among jurors.

This technique works. If it didn't, plaintiff attorneys wouldn't use it.

Choices and Consequences

Parties involved in nursing home litigation have three choices:

- Continue, believing that winning is possible
- Continue for a while, seeking a knockout
- Settle

These decisions aren't easy. Plaintiffs' counsel and clients have much to consider. When they believe that they're ahead, they'll exert all available sources of leverage. Settlement awards are often six or seven figures.

For family members, with limited financial risk due to contingency-fee arrangements with their lawyers, settling can mean a lot of money—for them.

Additionally, there's a psychological cost to trying a case. Family members aren't unscathed in litigation. While they may be surviving and sympathetic representatives of a patient's estate, they also stand to be beneficiaries of a decision against a nursing home. Their stories are important.

Relatives—in deposition or a courtroom—are asked about visit frequency and duration, grievances and complaints filed with nursing home leadership, reasons for not providing care to the patient at their own home, intra- and interfamily disputes, financial distresses involving any combination of family members, and rationale supporting the patient's continued stay at the nursing home.

This last item is consequential. Family members are frequently asked: "If things were so bad, why did you leave your loved one at the home?"

They sometimes respond, "Well, if I moved my mom (or dad), I wouldn't be able to keep an eye on them."

Or "I wanted to teach them a lesson."

In follow-up, lawyers will ask who exactly "them" is. Is "them" the nursing home, or their loved one?

For the defense, opinionators go beyond the nursing home and their legal representative. Owners, company executives, risk managers, in-house counsel, insurance carriers, third-party administrators—and more—will share thoughts and calculations on how best to proceed.

Following an event and throughout a suit's duration, opinions and decisions are fluid, influenced by what becomes learned and confirmed, and interpretation by parties on both sides.

When the laws are favorable to plaintiffs, and available information is damaging to the nursing home: *Advantage:* Plaintiff.

When the nursing home and its company has competent leadership and governance, an approach to care that supports providing best care possible, and representatives that can articulate this with confidence and conviction: *Advantage:* Defendant.

When there's no real advantage by either: *Pick 'em.*

Parties—believing they're ahead, behind, or even—have a decision to make:

Continue ... or settle.

ɕɔ

At trial, the weak are dared to defend themselves.

A nursing home's challenge, as defendant, is to distinguish between two competing questions:

Did the home *do something badly?* Or was the home *being bad?*

There's a distinction between the two. The former involves execution, the latter involves intent, or value structure.

Plaintiffs, especially when homes dare defend themselves, will argue *both* conditions apply, implying—or stating:

You did something bad. Because you are bad.

Unlike movie plots, the "good guys" do not always win. Even with a strong case and competent counsel, judges—and juries—can get it wrong.

Nevertheless, people—and companies—must live with themselves. Sometimes, they decide to fight and risk losing rather than surrender and take what's offered. The perceived insult of settlement is valued less than any injury of defeat.

Nursing homes and their companies will only dare to defend themselves when they have this in place:

- Superior defense counsel
- Competent, credible experts
- Competent, confident, and capable corporate representatives

Absent these, a nursing home is compromised. Victory is impossible. Settling is the sole path to survival. Plaintiff firms keep score, rating companies in each of these areas. In many cases, they are familiar with defense counsel, by firm or attorney reputation.

While defense counsel is relied on for their legal and technical excellence, their greatest value in defending the weak is in simplifying the complex for jurors, and extinguishing the fear and emotion that any combination of jurors might possess.

Serving as jury educators, they humanize people doing the work *that few want to do*, using logic to every instance where explanations of *who, what, when, where, why, and how* apply.

Their work as educators shouldn't end with juries. It *should* include educating a home or company on how best to improve or organize, thus mitigating—or preventing—repeat survey deficiencies or legal challenges.

For this to happen, however, it takes a willing nursing home or company interested in taking advantage of this instruction.

This is often easier said than done. And one reason why some things in nursing homes haven't changed over the past four decades.

A Two-Way Street

Superior work within homes, companies, and their defense counsel includes educational reciprocity—where providers become educators.

One assignment I had, in partnership with the senior vice president of professional services, was to achieve alignment and understanding among nearly one hundred defense attorneys, orienting each to the operating approaches taken by the company's several hundred nursing homes.

Aware of their disdain for PowerPoint presentations, and realizing that this opportunity might not recur during our tenure, materials shared with these important people involved a single slide.

One.

This is the complete text from the slide:

Top 10 Items We Need from Defense Counsel (2002)

10. *Know the organization you're defending.*
9. *Determine a safe method for two-way communication.*
8. *Develop working relationships with organization's leadership—especially regional VPs and nurses.*
7. *Tell us "how" more often than you tell us "don't."*
6. *Make an effort to learn "why" before you say "no."*
5. *Consider our size a positive, not a negative.*
4. *Stop feeling sorry for the executive directors (administrators) and directors of nursing.*
3. *When individual performance appears to be an issue, serve it up for discussion.*
2. *Enjoy your role as organizational educators.*
1. *If we are doing something stupid, tell us—we'll work to address it.*

During our hour together, Item #4—pitying the challenges of nursing home leaders—generated silent and audible reactions from attendees. Body language and facial expressions displayed visible discomfort.

Absent any questions, we addressed this directly, sharing views from our current and previous roles. With shared histories as nursing home administrators, we each identified with the role's demands and complexities, including supervising and developing a nursing partner.

Sharing these stories to these talented, committed defense attorneys, we highlighted the education backgrounds and total compensation packages for these positions—equaling or surpassing those of associates in their firms.

Audience postures shifted with each sentence.

Our parting thoughts could be summarized as:

- These leaders can rise to your expectations.
- And when they don't, it's OK to stick your foot up their asses.

Alignment accomplished. And for the next several years, this company and its nursing homes changed—for the better.

Settlements and Concessions

Patient care lawsuits, like other litigation—bankruptcies, divorces, estate challenges—eventually become a game of chess. The nursing home—or those with money on the line—realizes when it's time to concede and "tip over the King."

In the aftermath, *most* everyone gets paid. Plaintiffs, their counsel, and defense counsel. Experts, videographers, court reporters, and the state or municipality too.

Courtesy of the nursing home.

People with leverage or the power of the purse will *force* a settlement. Specifically, these parties work in this environment daily, measuring risk and expertly applying value to cases. Without emotion, they know when to hold 'em and when to fold 'em.

These parties include:

- **Representatives for the plaintiff.** Possessing the advantage, there's a dollar figure demanded, frequently coupled with knowledge of the insurance amount accessible to satisfy this demand.
- **Representatives for the nursing home.** Decision-makers include company executives and owners, in-house counsel, insurance carrier and third-party administrators, and outside defense counsel.

Settlements are most likely when insurance coverage sufficiently discharges a case without having to find other funding—e.g., cash or loans. This sometimes becomes a juggling act when multiple plaintiff firms have cases against the same nursing home, and coverage limits (or a per case basis or in the aggregate) are threatened. In these instances, plaintiff firms become willing to accept *something* rather than *nothing*—and *now* rather than *later*.

These dynamics result in interesting and difficult conversations.

These points begin explaining the *why* for litigation settlements. There are, however, deeper reasons *why* cases don't reach trial.

The power of the press is a deterrent to cases reaching trial. Trials can become emotionally charged, ripe for microphones and cameras, prior to or following a day's worth of courtroom activity.

Media-savvy plaintiffs' attorneys, politicians, and advocates have the ability to deliver daily damage to a home and company's reputation, resulting in an unmanageable environment. Their sound bites might not air on the nightly news (though they can), yet the advent of social media and media in the electronic age puts people on edge when things are unpleasant.

And trials are unpleasant.

ℭ

In addition to the powers of the purse and press, another massive reason for the weak choosing not to defend themselves: Companies—rather than nursing homes—are averse to questions about who does what, to whom, when, where, how often, and why.

Questions asked during cross-examination by *very* smart people provide witnesses *no quarter*. These are tests, graded by judges—who don't know or care too much about witnesses, or take kindly to responses like: "I'll have to get back to you on that."

Witnesses with poor preparation, poorer pedigree, or poorest processes ... *lose* in a courtroom.

In order avoid defeat, companies elect to not sit for these tests. For these companies, it's, *No questions, please. Let's just settle and move on.*

In several companies, it was common to provide executives with skill-building opportunities prior to their first (or next) experience as deponent or courtroom witness, through mock depositions or trials.

This investment of time, money, and attention, partnering with company attorneys or outside counsel, provided memorable, valuable experiences. These workshops helped me develop as a witness and benefit in future courtroom encounters.

I'll share a story when sponsoring this experience with a company later in my career resulted in much more than expected.

This nursing home company was smaller than other multilocation providers, with limited infrastructure and imagination. Dominated by family members, it had a lackluster litigation history, with owners and executives fatalistically embracing that nothing could be done to reverse field. Interestingly enough, competitors in the same state and markets appeared to have distinctly dissimilar experiences with their nursing homes.

Due to case history and inventory, and executive development needs, a mock deposition workshop was scheduled for the company's senior-most leaders. In advance, participants were requested to provide a complete résumé, so that questions could be prepared about their education and experience—or lack thereof.

This request rattled people.

Initial reactions among executives were private. Within days, behaviors were visible. Some worked at buffing up their histories, poll-testing newfangled titles for entry-level positions. Others manufactured compensatory explanations for their absence of industry experience prior to joining this company, or reconciling title inflation vagaries.

This behavior is common. People wrestle with telling their own stories. While life's elements make us unique, they create common ground among those who have changed schools, partners and spouses, jobs—by force or choice—and career paths. Nevertheless, glossing over, or excluding, gaps and imperfections can be an irresistible temptation.

Days before this workshop, an ashen-complexioned chief nursing officer entered my office doorway. Bracing myself for incredibly bad news involving one of the company's nursing homes or patients, I invited her to sit down.

After extended silence, she began speaking about the upcoming mock deposition workshop. Her body language indicated this experience wasn't going to be OK. Uttering a few near-incomprehensible sentences, I interjected, saying, "Slow down. What are we talking about here?"

She responded, "Dave, I don't have a bachelor's degree in nursing. I've never put my education on a résumé—only that I'm a registered nurse. I've never been asked about this, and wasn't when I was interviewed for this job."

This was a stunner. As this executive preceded me joining the company by nearly a year, I'd not known or expected this news. Her recruitment included multiple interviews with the company's CEO and HR leadership, repeated after each of the *three* times she declined this position's offering.

For a leader whose direct supervisory responsibilities included degreed nurses—bachelor's, master's, and advanced practice—oversight of physicians and pharmacists, and ownership for clinical strategies, operating guidelines, and expectations, this was an exceptionally wide educational gap between a C-suite executive (by title) and their charges, for which no real explanation sufficed.

This gap might have gone undetected for some time. At least until deposition or courtroom testimony.

This is one reason why companies will settle rather than defend themselves.

✥

Sadly enough, it doesn't end here. Mismatches in leadership's academic and educational preparation and their roles and responsibilities weakens a nursing home or company's ability to defend against legal challenges, as it raises questions of competence.

How then, do nursing homes and companies handle questions put to those without degrees?

Across today's industrial landscape, ambition, access to capital or debt, or a path paved by affinity can result in an instant CEO or C-suite executive.

No education required. A sponsor, cosigner, minority partner with a degree or two, and favorable, well-placed references that opens doors to those with money are the only requirements.

In the 2020s, this is fascinating.

Many of my ancestors were coal miners. There's a long line of people important to me that didn't don a cap and gown from junior high, let alone high school, college, or beyond.

Like others before and after, they had lifetime perfect attendance at the "School of Hard Knocks," creating lives—for themselves and their families—which are sources of never-ending pride.

With identical *life résumés* today, however, the likelihood of my ancestors accessing the working capital, line of credit, or mortgage with near zero down, and buying a nursing home—*or fifty*—is unfathomable. And a license to operate these homes, provided by state agencies—equally so.

Yet it happens. Achieving this entrepreneurial coup is celebrated among those able to create these self-employment opportunities.

These celebrations cascade throughout their organizations. Among nursing home companies that would prefer settling than defending themselves, organizational lineup cards at administrator, manager, director, VP, and C-suite roles are orchards of family trees littered with the weight of the academically, experientially, and educationally vacant resting on their branches.

At least until they can sell and get out, or convert their companies to a Real Estate Investment Trust (REIT), property leasing company, or some other entity that enables the spotlight to be shifted away from their deficiencies.

For these owners and CEOs, groupthink with heads of other nursing home companies serves as a proxy for continuing education. In traditional circles, we call this *happy hour, followed by dinner.*

Over time, echo chambers with colleagues emerge, resulting in a homogeneous blend of mediocrity as performance standards migrate to one method, or one vendor, displaying shades of the anticompetitive arrangements shared in earlier chapters.

Companies whose leaders possess these résumés and experiences are dogmatic in settling patient care litigation rather than having themselves or their work challenged.

This is easily understood. A skilled plaintiff's attorney would eviscerate an owner or CEO under these circumstances.

The question, asked by plaintiff's counsel—to those prone to discount academic preparation in this complex business, with caring for the most vulnerable at its center, and responsibilities for being a good shepherd of taxpayer dollars—*each day*—might be:

"Why *exactly* would you do this?"

Too harsh? No. Everything is in play when under oath. Counsel wouldn't stop here. They'd insist in learning how the leaders and owners with these life histories educated and developed their most valued workers—*and themselves*.

But this is simply storytelling. Settlement—and payment—would precede these questions.

ꟹ

In this industry of incentive-laden behavior, there's little wonder why these agents of change—the media, the legal profession, nursing home owners and operators, and for good measure, the government ... *haven't.*

While the rewards remain sufficient for these agents, the likelihood of behavioral and industrial change of scale is quite unlikely.

That is, of course, until people awaken, confronted with their own morbidity and mortality, realizing the necessity for change. By then, I fear it will be too little—and too late.

WHAT YOU CAN DO

Ask Questions About:

- The patient *bill of rights*
- How a home has changed and improved as a result of challenges experienced
- How adverse events resulting in patient injury are handled
- Responding and resolving grievances

Look for:

- Law firm-sponsored billboards, asking "Has Your Loved One Been Injured in a Nursing Home?"
- Internet history of the nursing home or company being featured in the media.

Listen to Yourself:

- Under what circumstances would you file a lawsuit?
- What would you expect to gain?
- Could you successfully endure direct- and cross-examination questioning from plaintiff and defense counsel?

VIII

BIG THINKERS, SMALL IDEAS

Working in a nursing home is a reality show. There's no artifice or spin. Successfully caring for people *and* business—for a shift, day, or week—is like winning a championship. Incredibly hard work and a little luck helps.

It takes years or decades to build skills and confidence to perform with competence and excellence. Work is complex and temperamental. Several disciplines require orchestration, each with shared *and* disparate goals, in a politically and emotionally charged environment, with slim margins separating life and death, comfort and pain, profit and loss.

Seemingly countercultural, given the industry's historical reputation for bloviating and begging, misplaced pride, myopia, and sloth, leaders might describe a nursing home's work as:

"You admit the patient, you take care of the patient, and you get paid for the patient."

People I've worked for described it:

"Fill beds, care for patients, hire and train best people, stay in compliance, and collect cash."

This approach is also found on the silver screen ... *Bull Durham*'s "Lollygaggers" scene sarcastically illustrates baseball's simplicity, as Skip, the Durham Bulls' manager, explains: "You throw the ball, you hit the ball, you catch the ball."[97]

Baseball professionals laugh at this description. And they should. The movie is a romantic comedy.

Same for nursing homes. Explaining the business model with, "You admit the patient …" or "Fill the beds …" is laughter-inducing.

While there are plenty of laughs and smiles in this reality show, a nursing home isn't a romantic comedy.

This chapter explores nursing homes' sobering and ever-growing challenges, solutions posed by leaders and influencers, methods by which they're derived, and parties assigned to execute, leaving you with a deeper understanding about the lack of change.

The Echo Chamber and Groupthink Narrative

In recent years, industry thought leadership has often been formed within an echo chamber. Common ownership—of homes and related-party entities—influences how companies organize, select vendors, define operating approaches and metrics, and determine value structures.

Substituting for creativity and originality, the echo chamber—via groupthink—opines, "If so-and-so is doing this, we should be too!"

Attend a few industry conventions, forgoing texting or catching up on emails, and listen.

As speakers, contributors, and attendees remark, groupthink emerges, like waves emanating from scorching hot asphalt.

Heads bob, like those kneeling over a water-filled tub full of apples on Halloween. The proliferation of private-equity ownership, explosion of related-party businesses, maniacal pursuit of high-acuity patients, and diminishment of RN staffing can be traced back to groupthink in the echo chamber.

Life within the echo chamber, among a homogeneous assembly of groupthinkers, is dangerous. Those with contrarian thoughts, challenging the status quo, risk being branded a rebel, an outcast—labels some avoid at all costs.

Across six decades in this business, rejecting groupthink within the echo chamber cost me. Sometimes, significantly.

Thankfully, one's work doesn't define them.

Echoed in publications, podcasts, and statements, these points briefly summarize the nursing home industry's current narrative:

- The public doesn't like us.
- The public doesn't trust us.
- The government beats us up.
- Too many beds are unoccupied.
- Too many positions for full- and part-time workers are unoccupied.
- If the government stopped beating us up, the public would trust us.
- If the public trusted us, they would like us.
- If the public liked us, our worker vacancies—and beds—would be occupied.
- If we don't get more money and relief—soon—it will be all over.

Brutally, some of these points are true. However, the government's role in the distress—and success—is an intellectual jump ball.

It's difficult to accept that governmental behavior is the universal determinant in the nursing home industry's destiny. This narrative ignores—or significantly narrows—the importance of markets, talent, strategy, and business cycles, instead placing responsibility at the feet of lawmakers, unelected bureaucrats, and taxpayers.

Allergic to Winning

Some nursing homes and their companies have been *loath to compete*. They found competition unsavory. Conversations about being best in market or vanquishing the field of competitors made managers and executives blanch.

To others it was a foreign experience. Never spending Friday nights or Saturday afternoons on playing fields, being pushed in classrooms, or driven to perfecting musical skills they were unfamiliar with playing to win.

Competing was a daily priority when I worked for public companies. Scorekeepers were everywhere. Analysts, investors, regulators, lawmakers, consumer advocates, institutions, and foundations kept their eyes on public nursing home company performance.

Patient care, people management, and business results were measured daily, weekly, monthly, quarterly, and annually. Scorekeepers did so obsessively.

Company role didn't matter. Awareness of metric-specific business unit performance was constant, as was company rank and comparisons among competitors within your market(s).

That defined the business of taking care of people and accepting taxpayer dollars.

Experiences were quite different in private nursing home companies. An obsession with being best in market was absent. Most owners were social and friendly with their peers. I'd not witnessed this collectivism before. More than an attitude, it was what one might envision in an arranged marriage.

Nursing home ownership reinforced this collectivism, as it included individuals (or their family's trusts) owning *other* nursing homes—and *vice versa*.

Further, these companies were inextricably linked by ancillary services relationships—performing *financial dialysis* on patients—whereby one home (or company) is contracted with a related-party company owned by another—*or vice versa*.

Sorting through the names and players in these arrangement types evoked this image:

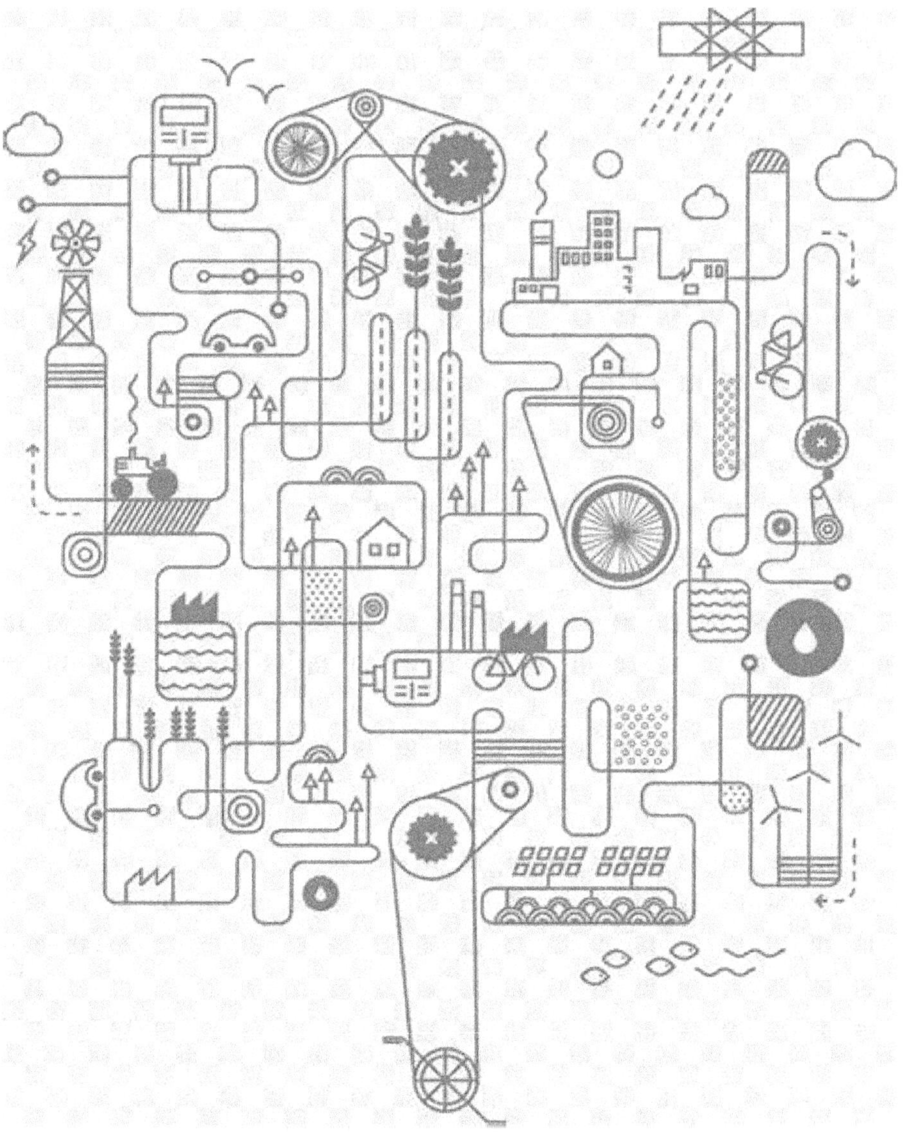

Little wonder these companies lacked competitive fire. Excellence—at the expense of another nursing home—was a self-inflicted financial injury. In this construct, there could be *no* losers. Losing was an injustice.

These ownership arrangements—in distinctly different companies—behaving collectively, infected strategic and tactical decision-making. This infection prioritized *never losing*, which differs from winning.

This activity, where neither side lost, was *playing to tie*.

As a result, nothing changed or improved. Public trust eroded. Taxpayer dollars burned. Patients and workers suffered the consequences.

Institutional Begging

Charles Dickens's classic, *Oliver Twist*, may be best remembered by this line: "Please, sir, may I have some more?" Remembering the book or movie, images of the dirty-faced orphan boy gripping the bowl beneath his chin, asking for more gruel, are indelible.

It exists within the nursing home world as well.

Begging. To lawmakers.

Executives assign trade association executives, lobbyists, and company representatives to carry empty bowls underneath their chins, asking for more. And they do it.

When lawmakers are approached for more—whatever *that* is—they want to talk to those working in the business. This was my experience.

I've *begged* with my own testimony. It was usually specific to Medicaid funding and proposed rulemaking for nursing homes in states where I lived and worked, as an administrator and territory manager. Years later, I participated in small group and one-to-one sessions with governors and key state and federal lawmakers.

In public hearings or private settings, I told stories and answered questions—about experiences, my employer, or other issues of which lawmakers and aides were curious. My work was to educate and inform.

Like witnesses in patient litigation cases, no one gets out unscathed. You're asking for things which empaneled inquisitors aren't inclined to give.

Lawmakers and aides do their homework beforehand, using the considerable resources at their disposal. They know things that you might have forgotten—or buried. As a result, one's credibility and history is judged aside their testimony.

When finished testifying, you're thanked for attending, and take the experience with you.

The Beggar's Playbook

***Money*, or funding, reimbursement, or appropriations,** is sought most fervently by Beggars. Their sentiment is, *pay us more, and everything will be OK.*

Bold requests aren't well received. Finesse is required. When testifying—or begging—I've strengthened pleas with employment statistics, payroll taxes paid, total patients served (and returned home), nursing homes under management, survey history, and other relevant facts as support.

And the bowl under my chin usually remained empty.

Money (MORE!) isn't the *only* thing Beggars have in mind. They ask for reduction or relief (LESS!) related to, or connected with, issues with financial implications. This grid of Beggar's Talking Points helps to MORE! or LESS! illustrate.

BEGGAR'S TALKING POINTS	
MORE!	**LESS!**
Money … from taxpayers.	**Regulation** … go look at someone else, OK?
People … from other industries and countries.	**Oversight** … trust me, we got this. Thanks.
Time … to delay what I don't like/want to do.	**Expectations** … got this too. Don't worry.
Trust … from all, earned or not.	**Disclosure** … you're on a need-to-know basis.

Respect … love us. You'll get old too.	**Scrutiny** … you shouldn't be looking at ME!
Flexibility … let us do our own thing.	**Bad Press** … go away, you just don't like ME!
Barriers … to all types of competition.	**Delays …** I thought I said we need it now!
Protection … of margins and valuations.	
Patients … many, and for as long as possible.	

This was the industrial version of The Beggar's Playbook during COVID, working to near perfection. Massive emphasis on MORE! and LESS!, anchored around other people's money (OPM), the nation's nursing homes benefited at a level equal to—or far surpassing—other industrial bailouts.

Lawmakers turned rainmakers, beginning with the CARES Act of 2020, followed shortly thereafter by the PPP.

In response, nursing homes *filled their bowls,* catching billions …

From various sources, including the Center for Medicare Advocacy, homes received this direct financial and nonfinancial support:

- Roughly *$21 billion* through the Provider Relief Fund[98]
- *$10.5 billion* in unsecured PPP loans—requiring no collateral or personal guarantee[99]
- Deferrals in previously scheduled Medicare cuts
- Expanded and accelerated advance payment programs

States also helped nursing homes *fill their bowls,* providing:

- Enhanced Medicaid rates for COVID-19 patients
- Incentives to create COVID-19-only nursing homes

- Across-the-board (ATB) adjustments in Medicaid rates to all homes
- Additional payments, including increased employee wage pass-throughs and other incentives

Payments were egalitarian. Poorly performing nursing homes were paid, as were those with exemplary performance history. Nursing homes living with massive survey and compliance issues were neither excluded nor penalized.

This is important. While the pandemic tilted the world, nursing homes that would have toppled, needing only a gentle push from *any* combination of government agencies ... *didn't*.

Trade association executives and lobbyists were near magicians. Lawmakers were merciful.

ဖ

Lawmakers also filled *bowls* with *stuff*. Nursing homes received crates of Personal Protective Equipment (PPE), bridging gaps in access, availability, competence, and creditworthiness.

County and State health departments visited homes, testing patients, and providing infection control technical assistance in arranging and monitoring patient populations. Some states went beyond, summoning the National Guard to provide care in homes unable to resolve staffing needs.

And there's more ...

Surveys were *suspended*, replaced with infection control walk-throughs. Homes were cited for technique and training breaches yet spared additional compliance and enforcement for over a year.

In its report, "States' Backlogs of Standard Surveys of Nursing Homes Grew Substantially During the COVID-19 Pandemic," the US Department of Health and Human Services, Office of Inspector General, indicated:

"Nationally 71 percent of nursing homes had gone at least sixteen months without a standard survey as of May 31, 2021."[100]

In its analysis, the Office of the Inspector General examined the percent of homes, by state, without a standard survey over the sixteen-month time frame, finding:

- Connecticut—96 percent unsurveyed
- Georgia, Oregon, Vermont, and Maryland—90 percent or greater unsurveyed
- 31 states at 70 percent or greater unsurveyed

Last, nursing homes were granted relief, and in some states—immunity—for civil litigation, except for willful misconduct or gross negligence.

For nursing homes, the pandemic was fruitful, MORE! or LESS!, including:

- Unprecedented increases in Medicare and Medicaid taxpayer funding
- Relaxed or deferred regulation, some which continues today
- Reduced threats to profitability through legislative support
- Zero visibility through prohibition of in-person family visits
- Substantial protections from patient liability claims

In short, *no nursing home was left behind.*

Compared to other industries, these results were superior, to the overwhelming satisfaction of many.

It Wasn't Enough?

An unanswered question to national and state trade associations and nursing home companies alike remains: *Where'd all this money go*?

No one's talking much. Instead, begging persists.

Please, sirs and madams, I want some more!—and less!

After receiving massive taxpayer largesse in 2020, the nation's nursing homes returned, carrying emptied bowls to their benefactors? *Why?*

Because the nursing home business became harder than people expected. Long-term survival would depend on competitiveness, efficiency, and developed, retained talent—contrarian rules of engagement to the collectivism of *there can be no losers.*

And they became scared. *Why?*

Because after a bailout of billions, workers traditionally electing for nursing home work—*now didn't*—and the breach of trust among everyday people who previously opted for nursing home care—*now wouldn't*—had resulted in an industrial failure to substantially restore prepandemic levels of patient census, mix, profitability, and cash flow.

Consequently, the American Health Care Association's (AHCA) April 2022 position paper, "Nursing Home Closures: By the Numbers,"[101] sounded the industrial alarm, stating:

"Nursing homes are struggling to recover from the pandemic and address a historic workforce crisis. Maintaining the status quo means *hundreds of nursing homes could soon close."* (emphasis added)

One inconvenient fact: In several prepandemic years, and 2019, hundreds of nursing homes *did close.*

This *has been* the status quo. Here's a condensed summary of nursing home closures from 2015–2021:

YEAR(S)	NURSING HOME CLOSURES (NATIONWIDE)
2015–18	556
2019	220
2020	145
2021	162

Source—AHCA

Furthermore, ACHA forecasted *400* nursing home closures "during the pandemic" in 2022. The grid below shows this forecast was too big, *by almost three-quarters*.

YEAR(S)	NURSING HOME CLOSURES (NATIONWIDE)
2022	108
2023	180
2024	176

Source: KFF[102]

This *forecast* could have been bad math or poor intelligence provided by member companies. Nevertheless, advancing this doomsday-like narrative and being this wrong was a bad look, leaving a welt—possibly permanent—on industrial credibility.

In 2020, lobbyists, owners, and industry executives scared the White House and Congress, and were rescued. With a different White House and congressional leadership in 2022 ... *not so much*.

Retrospectively, the endgame remains unclear. Was this industrial alarm sounded so:

- Regulators continued pumping the brakes on compliance matters?
- Congressional sympathy produced revised immigration laws?
- State and federal lawmakers filled their bowls, once more?
- Competition remained abated, thus protecting collectivism—a.k.a. *there can be no losers*?

It's hard to know.

What is known, and guaranteed, is that additional nursing homes will close. A decade's worth of history says so.

Physical plant age obsolescence, material market shifts, chronically poor patient care or financial performance, ineffective leadership, weak balance sheets, or the inability to effectively compete with alternatives available to patients and/or workers—guarantees nursing homes *will* close. *Every year.* Just like other businesses. *Every day.*

Nevertheless, nursing home closures are scary for companies, their owners, and related-party ancillary companies, vendors, and bankers.

Here's an example ...

An April 2023 *Skilled Nursing News* article, "'Tepid' Occupancy Recovery Continues with Flat Month for Post-Acute Care," reported Q1 2023 occupancy for nursing homes nationwide ranged from 72–75.5 percent. This meant many empty beds in some of the nation's nursing homes.[103]

With a nationwide average in the low-to-mid-seventies, nearly three years after the start of the pandemic, these performance results were scary.

Why? Because inside these statistics are nursing homes with very strong occupancies and others whose occupancy ... *sucked.*

For Some, It Was More Than Enough

Does all this spell trouble for the industry? *It doesn't seem so.*

Press releases and commentary from publicly held companies like The Ensign Group indicate strength and stability, achieving growth by capitalizing on the industrial misfires and misadventures.

Remarkably, they *returned* over $130 million in CARES Act bailout money—$110 million in August 2020,[104] followed by $23 million more two months later.[105]

Returned. Gave it back. Didn't need it. Remarkable, isn't it? While other US companies followed suit, I found no other nursing homes and companies that treated taxpayer money this way.

Industry brokers and deal makers didn't see troubling signs either. They believed that things would just get better.

Skilled Nursing News's June 2023 feature, "Why Skilled Nursing Deal Volume Could be 'Exorbitant, Voluminous' in Back Half of 2023," quotes Walker & Dunlop's managing director Mark Myers:

"While debt has been much more difficult to procure, and it is expensive, buyers of SNFs continue to have voracious appetites ... Buyers also have their *own ancillary companies that generate additional profits—sometimes as profitable or more so than underlying profits from SNFs."*[106] *(emphasis added)*

No doomsday-like narrative here. *Financial dialysis*—described in an earlier chapter—was a huge patient-centered catalyst for this optimism.

And yet, wait for it ... the begging continued. It will always continue.

Other People's People

Once the world tilted, people stayed at home. Workers didn't come back to work. This field remains barren today.

In some markets (and states), this dearth of labor creates barriers to access for the elderly and infirm, clogging hospitals with patients needing placement.

The narrative to solving these workforce deficiencies, advanced by industry and trade association leaders is ... *people from other lands.*

On its surface, this seems simple and expedient. If Congress and the White House were serious, bills would be passed, limits would be lifted, and problems would be solved.

If only it were this easy.

Through my lens, this is an intellectual and cultural surrender, the product of an uncompetitive industrial environment where winning—and changing—doesn't matter.

Additionally, this narrative—importing talent from countries—has described other professions and vocations for years. Only people from other lands will now do *these* jobs.

This proposed solution's arrogance is striking. A people problem, created in the US, should be assigned to other countries. As if they aren't suffering workforce deficiencies of their own.

In her September 2023 article, "Immigration Policies Must be Ethical and Equitable," Robyn Stone, DrPH, senior vice president of research at Leading Age, shared views of representatives from "younger, developing countries," on immigration as a solution to America's caregiver shortage while attending the Social Care International Workforce Summit in Glasgow, Scotland.

"Immigration is essentially, a *trade issue* between wealthy countries seeking to attract foreign-born workers and developing countries from which most immigrants hail ... out-migration of their citizens to developed countries is draining human resources and exacerbating workforce challenges at home. They warned us about ethical issues related to the *exploitation* of workers by those who arrange their migration and those who hire them."[107] (emphasis added)

Additionally, the World Health Organization's (WHO) report, *State of the World's Nursing 2020—Investing in education, jobs and leadership* (SOWN), indicates:

" ... current trends indicate thirty-six million nurses by 2030, leaving a projected needs-based shortage of 5.7 million."[108]

That's a lot of nurses. Among reasons for this projected shortage are an aging workforce, an undersupply of nursing educators, graduation rates failing to keep pace with demand, international mobility and migration, and worldwide underinvestment in the profession.

Solving the US nursing shortage via immigration might be a strategy ripe for rethinking. Worldwide competition for talented, caring scientists and specialists is, and will remain, massive.

The SOWN reinforces this point, stating in its "Ten Key Actions":

"Nurse mobility and migration must be effectively monitored and responsibly and ethically managed ... Countries that are overreliant on migrant nurses should aim toward greater self-sufficiency by investing more in domestic production of nurses."[109]

WHO's message to Beggars—stop relying on other countries. Get it together. Prepare, develop, and retain these valuable resources yourselves.

ఆ

I'll share this memorable, educational, and never-repeated experience involving other people's people (OPP). Here goes ...

Two nursing homes, a few miles apart, located in an affluent area, were experiencing incredible difficulties in attracting workers. Incumbents had been with both homes for years. Neither had "revolving door" turnover.

Economic and logistic imbalances further complicated matters. Like other affluent markets, frequent public transportation offerings were unavailable. Costs of living outpaced compensation models. Workers needed reliable transportation and the desire to commute long distances. Achieving this at scale was challenging. For many, including agency workers, it was too hard *or* not worth it.

Part of a multiyear effort between the company's HR and Recruitment departments involved bringing international workers to this market. Absent other practical and immediate alternatives, we decided to try it.

Workers arrived directly from Micronesia, a country comprised of hundreds of islands in the Pacific. With assistance from external agencies, candidates were screened and interviewed, securing work visas prior to arriving in the US.

A local hotel provided housing, with monthly rates negotiated, and rooms reserved for those coming to help.

Homes now had additional hands to help care for patients. For a while, this arrangement worked.

A short while.

Once work days ended, our visiting workers had limited options for their free time. They were in a foreign country, knowing only each other. As most workers were in their twenties and thirties, they did what people frequently do when on a trip ...

They partied. A lot.

The hotel contacted local and regional leadership about these peccadilloes. They were effectively managed for a while.

A short while.

To help bridge workforce gaps due to call-ins and illness, our visiting workers began piling up overtime, shortening available idle time, and accelerating the intensity at which they partied when able.

Nights became major blowouts, and the hotel management blew by the local and regional leadership, seeking people in the corporate office. Stories told by the hotel's exasperated general manager were like scenes from *Animal House*.

Days later, I visited the hotel and narrowly avoided being asked to buy it.

We shared an early goodbye with our visiting workers. This potential solution, though a failed experiment, was a valuable learning experience.

It's unknown whether this experience would be repeated at scale. Many of the risks, however, still remain.

Perfected matches in housing, language, food, religion, entertainment, transportation—will be difficult in markets where nursing homes seek other people's people. Chances for cultural alignment are likely stronger in major metropolitan areas, placing suburban and rural nursing homes—whose workforce issues are sometimes larger than their citified colleagues—at a deficit.

Even on a very small scale, this approach is likely to have material unintended consequences, as incumbent workers—that have hung tough through thick and thin—may perceive a double standard related to the attention paid to the *new kids on the block*.

Still, none of this will keep the Beggars from begging. A cautionary note to groupthinkers finding this a big idea …

Be careful what you wish for.

WHAT YOU CAN DO

Ask Questions About:

- Financial and nonfinancial help received during the pandemic
- Pay programs instituted during this time, and which remain
- Lessons learned from the pandemic experience
- Views on priority issues for state and national trade associations
- International workforce programming

Look for:

- Decision-makers and workers employed before 2020. Do they differ, compared to peers arriving afterward?

Listen for:

- Assigning responsibility to state and federal government—for *anything*
- Evidence of *begging*

IX

DISRUPTION IS INEVITABLE

Inuit legend suggests when elders no longer contributed to their communities, they were placed on ice floes and set adrift. In other cultures, especially when food was scarce, those viewed as a drain on precious resources risked being left behind.

It is unimaginable to confront this—*or any*—form of senilicide in the context of its time and culture whether it involves leaving someone in a cave, taking one to the top of a mountain, or tossing one from a bridge.

Isn't it?

It is, however, important to understand the significance of these practices in world history, as each exemplify the cultural value placed on the elderly (or infirm) and decisions regarding public and population health.

We're in the midst of a historic moment. And will be for a while.

Colliding social, political, and economic values may not invite families to pack their wares in darkness, leaving elders to spend final days in solitude, yet this collision will change the way we care for the elderly and infirm.

By the Numbers

Here are some facts to consider:

- **The US is growing old people.** The US Census Bureau reported the nation's age 65+ population (in 2020) at 55.8

million, or 16.8 percent. By 2030 "all baby boomers will be age 65 or older,"[110] with greater than eighty million, or more than 20 percent of the population, by 2040.[111]

- **Many old people are living alone.** In its "2020 Profile of Older Americans," the Administration for Community Living estimated nearly 15 million older adults lived alone, and less than 10 percent of these people lived in nursing homes in 2019.[112]

  In 2024, four years post-COVID, Americans living in nursing homes was approximately 1.2 million.[113]

- **Caring for these people is hard and expensive, and people don't seem to want to do it.** Previous chapters addressed these influencers, such as, staffing, workforce composition, competence, compensation, and the inability of nursing homes to recover workers lost since COVID.

  The expense, however, bears noting. CMS, in their July 2022 press release, "CMS Acts to Improve the Safety and Quality of Care of the Nation's Nursing Homes," estimated fiscal year 2022 *Medicare* spending to be *$33.5 billion*, and projecting another $1.7 billion in 2023.[114]

  Furthermore, they estimate, that in 2022, *Medicaid* long-term care services expenditures in the US were *$200 billion*.[115]

Nearly *$240 billion* ... in 2022. A number unlikely to tilt downward. *Ever.*

These are taxpayer dollars spent for institutional and home and community-based care *only*. Expanding to include all seniors, services, and associated taxpayer-funded healthcare spending, and this figure exceeds *$1 trillion* annually.[116]

If you asked patients, family members, and taxpayers, they'd probably tell you that the value received for the price being paid ...

Sucked.

A January 2023, Gallup article, "Americans Sour on US Healthcare Quality," shared these results from their annual Health and Healthcare survey[117]:

- Less than half (48 percent) now rate US healthcare quality as Excellent or Good.
- Americans' (72 percent) positive rating of their own healthcare quality is also a new low.
- Over half (56 percent) are satisfied with the total cost they have to pay for healthcare.

Where I attended school, 72 percent on anything wasn't Honor Roll material. In this context, Americans have scored American healthcare quality as far less than excellent.

For a price—healthcare spending, from all sources—reportedly at *$4.9 trillion* in 2023.[118]

Taxpayers paid a lot for a less-than-average grade. And the price continues to rise.

Looking Back, Then Forward

These facts, numbers, and sentiments are sobering. They'll gain momentum without change. Immediately, these questions arise:

- *Are the nation's nursing homes doing their very best?*
- *Will anything be different in five, ten, fifteen years from now?*

Affirmatively answering the first question is a really tough sell. In individual homes or companies, probably so. There are outstanding nursing homes, led by experienced, committed people, with intact workforces taking very good care of people, and delivering results to back it up. Generalizing across the industry, however, is a massive reach.

Over the next fifteen years, things will be very different.

Forty-eight years ago, on my first day working in a nursing home, upon entering a patient's semiprivate room, I found a man—a convicted felon—unable to return to prison, handcuffed to a bed, with roommates. No guard, cop, special precautions, or training. No specialized unit.

Just a guy, sicker than hell, shooting the shit while he watched me sweep and mop his floor. Today, this experience would occur in a distinct and highly secured location rather than in a community-based nursing home.

Thirty-five years ago, I began working for a company that demanded an edible garnish on every entrée. Familiar with the practice and purpose, my fourth skilled nursing employer was the first to enforce this standard.

Twenty-five years ago, I sided in arguments with colleagues about how to define and quantify patient care quality, frequently against those insistent on using satisfaction scores as the ultimate benchmark for quality. In time, metrics and standards for measurement accompanied key qualitative indicators, with aligned incentives which put the patient first.

Fifteen years ago, I spent three mornings a week with brilliant software developers and an expert-level wound care nurse, building a service that used clinically validated tools to identify patients at risk of pressure injuries, monitor healing, improve documentation accuracy and efficiency, and provide a suite of management reports to examine performance—presently and longitudinally—for one or several hundred—nursing homes.

Reeling in the years—across decades—is proof positive that things will be very different. History is undeniable.

These final chapters present thoughts about what is here and what possibilities await.

Disruption is at the heart of these possibilities, via:

- Medical momentum and breakthroughs
- Increasing insistence for self-determination
- Financing realities and awakenings
- Access contraction and market desertion

Medical Momentum and Breakthroughs

The first quarter of the twenty-first century has produced incredible advances in medical research, treatment, and technology. The list includes immunotherapy for cancer, HIV antiretroviral treatments, and medical cannabis, each finding its place among those living in nursing homes or avoiding placement due to their availability and application.

In the latter case, this is a victory. More wins await.

Today, Ozempic, Wegovy, Zepbound, and Mounjaro are part of daily conversations. Type "Ozempic face" into your browser and marvel at the transformation of formerly supersized entertainers and celebrities. Their body and facial changes cause "did they/didn't they" debates, especially among those not promoting a fitness center, protein drink, or ultimate marathon reality show.

These drugs, continuing critical mass momentum and public payor recognition, might change how type 2 diabetes and obesity are treated, worldwide, bringing sweeping change to the nursing home world.

This is easy to imagine. Today's nursing home patients suffer from these conditions—singularly or combined—with several generations awaiting, separated only by age, an acute event, or these chronic, debilitating conditions advancing.

With thanks to Novo Nordisk and Eli Lilly, future nursing home candidates might never reach waiting lists. Treatment options could radically change individual health trajectories, mitigating or eliminating concomitant risks associated with diabetes and obesity, and prolonging—or staving off—any need for admission.

And in doing so, reduce the likelihood for treatments like kidney (and financial) dialysis.

Note: I'm an investor in Eli Lilly.

Regardless of firm or drug, these options will have a ripple effect in delaying or reducing the incidence of traditional primary and secondary nursing home diagnoses, including heart attack, heart failure, stroke, chronic kidney disease, hypertension, urinary incontinence, and depression.

Delay these serious health conditions by one, five, ten years, or more, and the demand for nursing home beds could be impacted considerably.

On any given day, less sick people, sick of being sick, means less nursing home beds needed.

In a broader context, the effect on weight and health could reduce postsurgical nursing home stays related to orthopedic procedures—like *hip and knee replacements.* Though lessened in recent years, these short-term stays could slow to a trickle.

Imagine the possibilities. According to the Johns Hopkins Arthritis Center, "being only ten pounds overweight increases the force on the knee by 30–60 pounds with each step." [119]

As someone whose knees have been surgically repaired multiple times, it's easy to envision people forgoing these procedures due to easing the force routinely placed upon their joints and reducing chronic pain.

Certainly, there's more to learn about the long-term implications and improvements and how patients can access treatment affordably. Additional research will bring refinements, and additional success stories will stimulate conversations about broad-based financing and expanded access. Employers and insurers may play a leadership role in this effort, with state and federal programs to follow—or vice versa.

It's easy to argue that, in individual cases, risks and side effects outweigh benefits. People are taking these risks, as it seems that any medicine accomplishes only *one* of two things:

You will feel better.

You will live longer.

But you only get one of these things to happen. *And you get to choose which one.*

The significant health implications of obesity, diabetes, and their affiliated comorbidities, and the availability of these treatment options now let people work with their physicians to examine and choose their preferred path.

Deciding between the risks of nausea, diarrhea or constipation, or other gastrointestinal discomfort, or continued disability and immobility, stroke, an accelerated path to death, or constant, chronic pain is serious business.

These options now give people a chance to choose.

ග

Pain and suffering is overrated. Yet, lots of people endure it.

The CDC, in its April 2023, report "Chronic Pain Among Adults—United States, 2019–2021," estimated "50 million adults in the United States experienced chronic pain (i.e., pain lasting ≥ 3 months) in 2016."[120]

Fifty million. The population of Texas and New York, combined.

Additionally, "During 2021, an estimated 17.1 million persons experienced high-impact chronic pain (i.e., chronic pain that results in substantial restriction to daily activities)."[121]

We know people who fit in one of these categories. And we know how they treat their pain.

Some take the old-fashioned approach—*if it hurts, don't do it.* Or, a long-standing, though newer approach—*better living through chemistry*, using street, prescription, and over-the-counter drugs for relief. A can or bottle may ease their pain—sometimes all day, most times every day.

Eventually, their pain is shared with us—socially, financially, emotionally, or physically.

Others manage pain differently, consistently, and effectively. While polarizing, it returns us to the 1960s and 1970s, or the "Reefer Madness" movement of the mid-1930s.

I am "reefer-ing" to cannabis.

Legal for medical use, per The Cannigma, in forty-one states, Washington, DC, and Puerto Rico, and decriminalized in more than over twenty, the nation's map will eventually "go green," supporting cannabis use, medically and recreationally.[122]

When? I don't know. I do believe, however, that states currently abstaining won't hold out indefinitely.

Why? Tax revenues lost to neighboring states will be intolerable. Eventually, public sentiment will weaken and crater. Like Sunday alcohol, state lotteries, casino gambling, and online betting, cannabis will become mainstream everywhere.

Federal lawmakers will legalize it too. For the same reason.

The money is simply irresistible.

For now, those able to legally manage their pain with cannabis—will and do—and those that can't—will and do ... *too.*

While people await universal recognition and broad underwriting of palliative care by taxpayers, they're not waiting for lawmakers and policymakers. Those in pain *now* reach for solutions, including cannabis, to feel, function, and live better.

As an oil or gummy, baked in brownies, vaped, or rolled and smoked, people of all ages and conditions have moved to that which grows from the soil. Pain is lessened. They feel better. And tell me so. Simplifying the complex, without trivializing the serious, I ask:

Does it work? Almost always, for pain and anxiety.

Does it need to be taken every day? Every day they need to.

Are you worried about being impaired? Without it, they are badly impaired.

This is what feeling better sounds like.

In addition to mitigating pain, cannabis is being used to reduce suffering. Jazz Pharmaceuticals' Epidiolex was the first FDA-approved prescription of cannabidiol (CBD) to treat seizures associated with a series of diseases, and Cardiol Therapeutics has two products in therapeutic development, one to treat recurring pericarditis and acute myocarditis, and another intended for use in heart failure. Though results in the latter cases remain pending, and scores of clinical trials end without breakthroughs, these pursuits are causes for optimism.

If time travel were real, we could forge ahead, like Bill and Ted did in their "Excellent Adventure" and know with certainty.

In the same vein, we could travel backward, imagining the life for those in pain who could rub something on their arm, leg, shoulder, or back, eat something smaller than a Swedish Fish, or spark up without fear of contamination—or worse—and understanding the net effect of these existing interventions.

Opioids might never have been necessary. People might have been more independent and functioning for much longer than their histories, never needing a nursing home.

ᔓ

Leading off with medical momentum and breakthroughs for obesity, diabetes, and chronic pain might cause readers to go ... *meh.* Why? Because while they effect many nursing home patients, everyday people might not identify either in their top five.

Why? People don't equate *death* or premature aging with these diseases and conditions.

Understandably so. Americans are conditioned to shake off pain, spitting on a finger and making the sign of the cross, or taking two Advil and getting back out there. Diabetes, as a disease, is neither widely understood nor frequently discussed. Largely invisible, it's rarely witnessed, except for people who go to dialysis or have limbs and digits amputated.

And obesity ... isn't openly discussed. Too hot to handle. Talking about it might result in fat shaming. Not OK.

No, these diseases or conditions wouldn't be top responses among those surveyed. This one would: Alzheimer's.

People understand this. They know someone whose life was impacted by Alzheimer's disease.

It is scary. Once diagnosed with Alzheimer's, friends and family know the clock's ticking, counting down to when the person loses touch with themselves and others, and eventually dies.

People understand this—*immediately*.

Why? The CDC, in "Data Brief 492. Mortality in the United States, 2022," placed Alzheimer's #7 among causes of death, nationally, involving roughly 120,000 people annually. This ranking was the same in 2021, displaced from the #6 hole by COVID, to which it will likely return.

Ahead of Alzheimer's (excluding COVID) are familiar causes, including heart disease, cancer, accidents, stroke, and lower respiratory diseases. Finishing off the top 10, diabetes ranks eighth, kidney disease ninth, and chronic liver disease and cirrhosis is tenth.[123]

These causes, while attention grabbers, are not easily identifiable. Signs are invisible, including behaviors. Think about it—can anyone accurately identify the future victim of a fatal car accident among Wal-Mart shoppers?

The Alzheimer's Association's "2024 Alzheimer's Disease Facts and Figures Report: Executive Summary" provides more:

- *6.9 million* Americans age 65 and older have Alzheimer's, with another *200,000* Americans under 65.
- The total cost of caring for people with Alzheimer's and other dementias in the US (from all sources) is expected to reach *$360 billion* in 2024, *with another* nearly *$350 billion* in unpaid caregiving provided by family and friends in 2023.
- The total lifetime cost for someone with dementia approximates *$400,000*, with *70 percent* of costs borne by family caregivers in the forms of unpaid caregiving and out-of-pocket expenses.[124]

This is why people understand this disease, and others like it. Signs of Alzheimer's and related dementias are visible—physically, functionally, and statistically. Maybe not during early stages, though later they're hard to ignore.

On a macro scale, Alzheimer's isn't being ignored, which is why possibilities remain causes for optimism.

In 2011, Congress passed, and the president signed, Public Law 111-375, the National Alzheimer's Project Act (NAPA), appropriating money to accelerate research and treatment "that would prevent, halt, or reverse the course of Alzheimer's."[125]

Prevent, halt, reverse ... *Fighting* words.

This Act signified, like only cancer and AIDS beforehand, that work directed at Alzheimer's—through the NIH—would bypass traditional budgetary review processes and receive annual congressional support via a Professional Judgment Budget directly submitted to the Secretary of Health and Human Services' (HHS) Advisory Council on Alzheimer's Research, Care, and Services.

By the looks of it, We, The People are throwing money at it. Take a look at the funding history since 2014, with figures courtesy of the Alzheimer's Association-sponsored Alzheimer's Impact Movement:

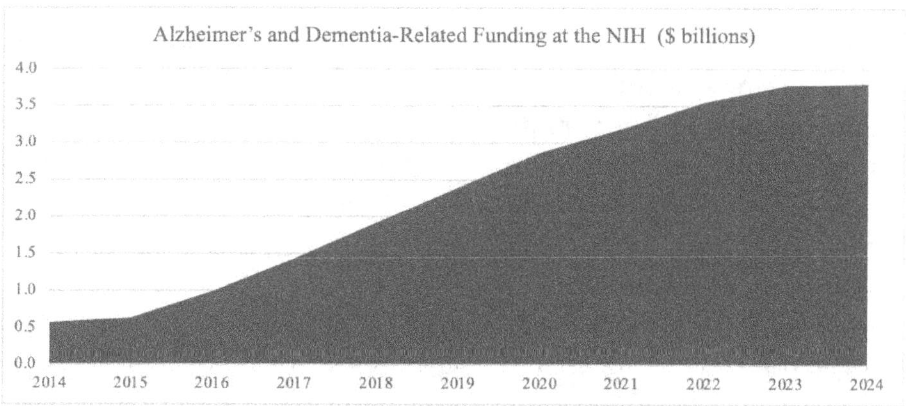

This is big money. The investment appears to be generating returns. In his May 2022, blog, "NAPA at 10: A decade of Alzheimer's and related dementia research progress," Dr. Richard J. Hodes, Director of the National Institute on Aging (NIA) at the NIH, shared:

- Researchers have identified more than *seventy* associated genetic areas, compared to ten genes ten years ago, and *four* genes twenty years ago.
- Researchers can now use brain imaging methods of lab tests to diagnose people living with the disease.
- NIA supported more than *400* clinical trials for Alzheimer's and related dementias, compared to *38* in 2015.[126]

This raises hope for bigger things ahead. As Congress recently extended NAPA through 2035, researchers have plenty of running room for discovery.

Results for previously marketed Alzheimer's-related discoveries have been mixed. With props to Drugs.com for their historical development timelines, the FDA granted accelerated approval in June 2021 to Biogen's Aduhelm. After a two-and-a-half year run, absent CMS payment approval, Biogen pulled the plug on it in January 2024.

Why? Doesn't matter. People at Biogen learned something. This learning mattered.

See, a year before discontinuing work on Aduhelm, Biogen—in partnership with Eisai—received FDA-accelerated approval of another drug, Leqembi, whose clinical trials demonstrated a *slowing* of the disease's progression.

Six months *later*—in June 2023—Leqembi received traditional FDA approval, and payment approval by CMS and the US Department of Veterans Affairs.

This is a victory, not a loss. *Why?*

Slowing down Alzheimer's disease and related dementias is an incredibly good thing.

Every day matters. Giving people an extra day—of cognition, memory, function, and sociability—is one *more* they might spend home with their families, and one *less* in a nursing home.

With history as guidance, strides in cancer and AIDS research—worldwide—prove that big things can happen when time, money, and talent is invested.

Want to bet against America playing a starring role in eventually preventing, halting, or reversing the course of Alzheimer's? I surely don't.

ꟹ

To this point, these future possibilities are reactive. Like everyday living, when something happens, something else happens in response. A successful response is usually a function of time, skill, resources, or—luck.

Luck frequently runs out. So can time. But using time differently, to get ahead of something that might happen, prepares people well for when it does.

The final element in medical breakthroughs we'll explore involves getting ahead of something before it might happen. In this case, using genome engineering or altering the sequence of one's DNA—the biological fingerprints that make us ... *us*.

This work is known as CRISPR-based therapies directed at eliminating, modifying, activating, or replacing a person's genome(s).

Or ... treating diseases with a genetic cause. The goal is to get ahead of these diseases, and doing it as early as possible.

To consider the possibilities here requires rolling the clock back a few years.

In 2020, scientists Jennifer Doudna and Emmanuelle Charpentier received the Nobel Prize in Chemistry for, per www.NobelPrize.org, "discovering one of gene technologies sharpest tools: the CRISPR/Cas9 genetic scissors."

This fascinating story and description of their work have two statements worth knowing, the first of which is:

"This technology has revolutionized the molecular life sciences ... contributing to innovative cancer therapies and making the dream of curing inherited diseases come true."

Here's a shorter version: "Genetic scissors: a tool for rewriting the code of life."

The important scientific, ethical, legal, and societal implications associated with work of this magnitude fail to dim "the dream of curing inherited diseases come true." The possibility of curing acquired diseases before they shorten, chronically impair, or end a person's life is simply ... mind-blowing.

As debates continue, worldwide efforts by CRISPR-focused companies are devoted to illnesses and conditions, including kidney disease, heart disease, obesity, cancer, leukemia, diabetes, sickle cell anemia, childhood blindness, Down's syndrome, infections, viruses, and neurological diseases—like Alzheimer's and Parkinson's.

It's the top of the first inning for genome engineering. Combining research-based results with the power and speed of machine learning, the real possibilities are likely still ahead. With sustained momentum, medicine will increasingly become *specific to the person*, rather than *specific—or general—to the disease.*

Like Alzheimer's, time, money, and talent is being invested in CRISPR-based therapies. The top five CRISPR companies, based on market capitalization, are reflected below:

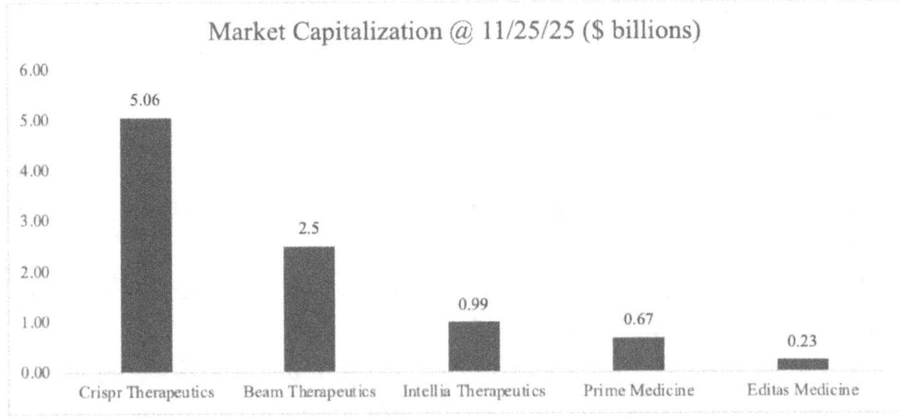

Source: www.companiesmarketcap.com

It's an industry large enough to get—and keep—people's attention.

Note: I'm a shareholder in Editas Medicine, Beam Therapeutics, and CRISPR Therapeutics.

As work evolves, the long-term impact on nursing homes might be more profound. By *getting ahead and doing it as soon as possible,* people could enjoy days, months, or years with improved—or superior—health, never needing to spend a day in a nursing home.

I hope those days come soon.

Increasing Insistence for Self-Determination

***Self-determination* is a term that people love—or detest.** Quoting Frank Sinatra, people view self-determination as "All, or nothing at all ..."

You can relate. Teenagers love the freedom to choose. And their parents—maybe not so much.

Fast-forward several decades, and you'll find identical dynamics among parents and children—*in reverse*. Parents dig in, with the intent of holding on to the last vestiges of their liberty, even at the risk of injury.

Like New Hampshire's state motto—"Live Free or Die." Or ... for Bruce Willis fans, *Live Free or Die Hard*.

Among former teenagers—now adult children who've accumulated their own life's baggage—urges sometimes tilt, infantilizing parents, discouraging them from things that might look awkward, lack precision, or appear unsafe.

Like what? Making coffee, slicing *anything*, doing laundry, putting *anything* in a microwave, using a computer, arranging for time outside the home with *anyone* for *any reason*, and sharing *any* thought, remark, or viewpoint held or said since the day these adult children were born.

Seen *any* of this? If you haven't—*yet*—OK. This too may happen to you.

When adult children infantilize their parents, *their makers* dig in deeper, further escalating risks. Parents, out of spite or to demonstrate "they're capable," will hide things and experiences from adult children, sometimes taking it too far—resulting in injury, illness, or worse. This is the *fun* in *dysfunction*.

The irony of this experience is that it's highly likely to be repeated when these adult children—insisting on infantilizing their parents today—become geezers, courtesy of their own adult children. More *fun* for them.

Geezers without kids are relieved of this experience, though relief is quickly replaced with other potential risks, like loneliness and isolation.

Remember, Bette Davis said … "Getting old isn't for sissies."

☙

While unavoidably true, disruptors are gaining traction, and likely to give contemporaries, elders, and future generations a chance to embrace the final lines from a poem familiar to many …

"Do not go gentle into that good night.

Rage, rage against the dying of the light."

Welshman Dylan Thomas never made it to Geezer Nation, dying shortly after his thirty-ninth birthday. Instead, he left this sage advice to the living. These next disruptors, many you are likely familiar with, will provide people the opportunity to extend their independence and maintain self-determination.

They require no technological advances. Only the time and touch of another person. And will massively challenge the status quo.

Present today on a microscale, each possess commonalities, polarizing everyday people. One of these needs a little help from friends to become mainstreamed. The other, however, likely requires overcoming generations of fear, a commitment to major-league consumer education, and an appetite among public policymakers.

For my memory's length, an unhealthy tension has existed within the value structure toward sick people. The tension—among practitioners, interested observers, and opinion-makers—demands respect and dignity for the patient, and places a premium on the stoicism, heroism, and the incredible suffering people endure for years, months, days, or minutes before death.

For those unfamiliar, the path to death for a person with a chronic illness—or pain—is very undignified. *It's not pretty.* When mind and body are no longer synchronized, the physiological and behavioral results are unimaginably undignified.

It's not like seeing an injured athlete, downed on the field with a broken bone, where the cart comes out and minutes later, they raise a thumbs-up gesture to the crowd, followed by full-throated chanting and applause.

That's not it. It's heart-wrenching, ripping pieces from your soul while you watch across the minutes, days, months, or years. Yes, unfortunately people endure this agony for years.

Many.

When it involves people that you love, three thoughts race through your head:

- This might be the most frightening thing I've ever seen, and I wish it weren't happening.
- This pain and suffering is intolerable.
- Please, make this end quickly … for everyone.

While the person's pain is managed ineffectively—meds aren't working, thoughts and emotions are on overdrive, they're scared—sometimes they know *exactly* what will make them feel better, and it doesn't always have a diagnosis code.

People who mattered to me, while suffering in pain, have asked …

- Hold my hand.
- Rub my back.
- Hold me close.

- Tell me a story.
- Sit by me and don't leave.

Some people can't ask. It's too hard. They simply won't do it. Or an even bigger tragedy, they don't have a person to ask.

After the suffering ends, no matter how long it might have taken, platitudes by those left behind can be endless. Read a few posts on social media or attend a few memorial services and this quickly becomes apparent.

People do this for their own reasons. This is how *they manage their pain.*

Palliative Care

Too often, however, the departed didn't have their pain managed well enough. They lived in fear and agony for too long. If interviewed from their graves, they might ask their mourners …

What the hell are you crying about? Didn't you see what was happening to me?

Many people—and physicians—are unskilled at everything about death and dying. The experience is considered too painful. Yet there is a movement afoot specifically and intentionally designed to help manage pain—for the patient and everyone connected—called palliative care.

Contrary to convention, palliative care is a specialty. Distinctly different from other specialties, as oncology is from cardiology.

Why? Becoming expert at treating pain and suffering isn't an online certification program for doctors. The approach is to treat the *entire* person, beyond the disease or condition. Learning how, then doing this, is hard.

Why? Every person is different. In pain tolerance. Communication skills. Ability to receive and interpret information when they hurt. Because this specialty is person-specific.

Palliative care experts in medicine, nursing, pharmacy, social work, nutrition, therapies, and direct caregiving need to learn and know about what matters, such as advanced care planning, medication management, care coordination—for example, with specialists like oncologists, cardiologists, pulmonologists—counseling, and effective patient communication.

It sounds like a lot, and it is. This helps define the—as yet—fully undefined.

Though available and provided today, through several Programs of All-Inclusive Care for the Elderly (PACE) across the nation, palliative care is neither well known nor understood. Physicians, nurses, nursing home workers, and everyday people might have heard the term yet wrestle to explain with confidence.

An incredible opportunity awaits.

A July 2021 study, published in the *Journal of the Advanced Practitioner in Oncology*, "Early Palliative Care of Oncology Patients: How APRNs Can Take the Lead,"[127] measured knowledge depth by surveying advanced practice registered nurses "at a large Midwest teaching hospital."

Study results indicated, "93 percent of respondents understood that Palliative Care is appropriate for all seriously ill patients" and "most of the respondents had a good grasp of symptom management."

Less encouraging findings included, "only 38 percent understood that Palliative Care and aggressive treatment can be offered simultaneously."

Last, and stunningly is that "the survey found that 100 percent of respondents felt that the extent of the disease should determine pain management."

This is research-speak for the patient ***gets*** pain management when the nurse practitioner *decides* that *they are sick enough* to get relief.

The unhealthy tension within the value structure toward sick people will eventually be resolved. This survey alone is cause for optimism. Important people are talking, listening, and learning.

It's premature to extrapolate these results across the spectrum of US healthcare providers. Years of experience, including my mother's final days, lead me to presume that We, The People suffer from a dearth of public and medical community awareness about the possibilities of palliative care.

Why? Because insurers—private, Medicare, Medicaid—*may pay some* for palliative care. In this case, "some" is a technical term. Payment for palliative care is likely be "baked into" other services already covered by these insurance programs, rather than a distinct, stand-alone service line or defined benefit.

Why? Because there's fog in viewing palliative care as a *specialty*, and institutional ignorance of its practical, financial, and patient care benefits.

But that's today. Treasure can't stay buried forever.

Studies and testimonials indicate that palliative care, delivered before and during a patient's end-of-life experience, saves money, reduces hospitalizations, and enhances quality of life—including the ability to remain at home. Search "benefits of palliative care" and there's content sufficient to improve one's knowledge.

Someday, palliative care will become well understood and frequently utilized. That day will likely coincide with widespread positive public and professional sentiment, resulting in payment infrastructure, discipline-specific quality standards, and respect for small- and large-scale data sources validating the value proposition of this little known and underutilized specialty.

When widely adopted, like current PACE participants, people will possess an option to institutionalization, remaining at home, preserving self-determination—while their chronic pain is actively managed—*regardless of the extent of the disease.*

The World Health Organization defines palliative care as a process that "intends neither to hasten nor postpone death."

Arguably, this definition is perfect. Achieving it, however, is quite imperfect.

As a provider and observer of care, across many years and patients, the social, ethical, emotional, and professional considerations are profound. Intending neither to hasten nor postpone death—while virtuous—can be entirely dependent on the lens through which the process is viewed.

A practice testing this virtue is palliative sedation. Occurring in end-of-life care, this practice involves introducing medication so that pain that is otherwise unmanageable can be, without rendering the patient unresponsive.

While this practice doesn't accelerate death, through sedation, the patient—no longer receiving nutrition or hydration—eventually cedes to a terminal condition. It's important to distinguish between the *person*, who by definition of receiving treatment by a hospice provider is terminally ill, and the *method* by which excruciating pain is managed.

As a son who has experienced this with his own mother, distinguishing between *person* and *method*, regardless of provider type or care environment, challenges all mental and emotional activity occurring between your ears and heart.

Nevertheless, I am grateful—for Mom and me—this practice exists.

Through one lens, it's arguable that while palliative sedation may not hasten death—it doesn't postpone it either. Conversely, because this treatment—intended to reduce a person's pain and suffering—affects a person's respiration, it can be argued that it indeed hastens one's death.

Quite a topic for a bioethics lecture.

This next, fiercely debated lifestyle disruptor will provide people with total control right up to their life's final seconds.

In movies depicting WWII spies or secret agents, and the go-to equalizer to keep "bad guys" from securing valuable intelligence, is for heroes to chomp on a cyanide pill. James Bond, Ethan Hunt, and so on ... Their premature dates with death, placing country—or mission—before self, would be celebrated.

Yet off the silver screen, this act of self-determination is considered ignoble—questioned, criticized, or mocked. To some, suicide is condemned as a moral sin.

Conflicts involving fear, selfishness, and compassion depend on your closely held values, including self-determination.

In much younger days, I wrestled massively with these conflicts. I haven't for years.

Why? Because the FACES Pain Scale, measuring from 1–10, doesn't always effectively assess one's pain. Especially when it's not easily visible, or the person in pain is tired of talking about it—or having it measured.

In some situations, tired people—in pain and suffering—are seeking help. If you will, some *assistance*.

And they are getting it. Providing people more control over their bodies and the quality of their lives is gaining momentum. In time, the lifestyle demand for enhanced self-determination will have a steamroller effect.

There are too many judicial precedents, financial and economic barriers, and stories of real and incredible suffering keeping this from becoming a national reality.

Medical aid in dying (MAiD)—otherwise known as assisted suicide—is an end-of-life option for eligible patients to self-administer a medication prescribed by a physician to hasten their death. This option currently exists in eleven states, plus Washington, DC.[128]

During 2025, New York's State Assembly and Senate passed MAiD legislation, signed into law in February 2026. It now joins California—another historical bellwether in driving legislative change—in codifying a person's right to self-determination.

Those interested in learning more about the history and international effect of MAiD—and its legal, legislative, ethical, and practical elements—

should consider reading Dr. Stefanie Green's book "This Is Assisted Dying—A Doctor's Story of Empowering Patients at the End of Life."

Across the books I've read—ever—this is among the most impactful about *living and loving*. It should be required reading for anyone in healthcare or medicine.

Changing specialty from maternity, Green writes extensively of her experiences in Canada, from the first days of helping people access help with MAiD, to her leadership in forming and serving as President of the Canadian Association of MAiD Assessors and Providers.

Among the many poignant thoughts shared by Green, this confirmed that momentum will continue unabated:

"... after a global AIDS epidemic, or perhaps due to a generation of aging baby boomers, there was a rise in the effort to improve the quality of life remaining instead of focusing on extending life at any cost—there was a growing interest in reclaiming death and dying through good palliative care and, in a number of jurisdictions around the world, through assisted dying."[129]

Green's review of the legalized assisted dying programs in Netherlands (physician-centric), the US (voter- and ballot-centric), and Canada (patient-centric) belie value structure differences which dilute or fortify one's ability to *own* their bodies, and destinies.

The most encouraging trend is that action is occurring at the state, rather than federal, level, allowing voters to decide locally.

Cultural, religious, and social considerations will likely remain intensely personal, allowing people to accept or reject anything and everything about this option.

As it should be.

Choose it or not, the *right to choose* is what matters.

Financing Realities and Awakenings

Money makes the world go 'round. Though an uncomfortable topic, today's money matters are making disruption unavoidable.

Among the old *or* sick, money is frequently in the front of one's mind. Among the old *and* sick, physical, mental—and financial—health are inextricably linked. Prices, premiums, and copays. Coverage and eligibility. Home- and community-based programming. Utilities and insurance. Owning versus renting, Moving or staying put. Inflation and access. Income, cash flow, and debt.

One's past directly influences the present. Earnings histories and savings rates. Pensions and Social Security. Early retirement, or work until death. IRAs and 401(k)s. Mortgage-free living, paying down a home equity line of credit, or a reverse mortgage. Long-term care insurance—*or not.*

And the present directly influences the future. Family member interest and support and their capacity to continue. Or the reverse—providing continued support for adult children, or grandchildren. Taxes of all types. The state of one's State. The health of the Nation. Medicare, Medicare Advantage. Medicaid.

If you're directly or tangentially interested in taking care of another, or pondering how best to exercise and retain your own self-determination, understanding money, individually and collectively, on a micro and macro scale, is essential. Otherwise, you can hurt someone you love—or yourself.

Political affiliation and generation aside, these numbers from www.usdebtclock.org—are constantly growing, and sobering:

US National Debt	$36,235,141,566,282
US National Debt Per Person	$104,873
US National Debt Per Household	$271,620
Total US Unfunded Liabilities	$123,303,867,354,555
Social Security Unfunded Liability	$15,115,285,325,321
Medicare Unfunded Liability	$79,039,382,303,521

Prescription Drug Unfunded Liability	$19,946,359,353,561
National Healthcare Unfunded Liability	$9,202,840,372,152
Total US Unfunded Liabilities Per Person	$356,869
Total US Unfunded Liabilities Per Household	$924,290
US Population	345,515,865

These figures are polarizing as well. Washington DC lawmakers share competing viewpoints by the hour. Their comments range from "this is a clear and present danger" to "nothing to see here," resulting in *FUD*—Fear, Uncertainty, and Doubt. While jousting ensues, questions multiply about the form, function, and future of Medicare and Medicaid, and the impact of legislation on what and how much is paid, for whom, and for how long. The recently passed *"One Big Beautiful Bill" Act* is evidence of this.

The nation's governors are especially impacted as individual states are dependent on congressional and White House decision-making. Since states can't print or circulate their own currencies, these fifty elected problem-solvers are limited in their menu of potential options and solutions.

As a result, states must take care of their business through fiscal policy, coordinating tax policy and programming to achieve intended goals. While simplistic, this summary of state-specific economics helps illustrate the limitations governors experience as they balance and manage political, practical, and party demands and figure out best ways to balance Medicaid dollars for institutional and home and community-based programming. Programs (or payments) that fall to *the cutting room floor* mean more out-of-pocket payments from everyday people—or simply doing without.

❧

Feel like this is all too much? Hell, yes indeed, it is. Nevertheless, this current state—within households, families, cities, states, and the

US of A—leaves people with no alternative but to follow the money on a micro and macro scale in determining what is best for themselves and ones they love.

As we've touched on some of the nation's financial indicators, it's worth highlighting just *one* at the state level. *Why?* Because inevitably, old, sick, or old *and* sick people will likely be forced to take notice.

From the November 29, 2023, www.gobankingrates.com article, "US States With the Most (and the Least) Debt"[130] *indicated:*

States with *lowest* Debt to Asset Ratios:

- Idaho 10.68 percent
- Alaska 14.68 percent
- Utah 15.93 percent

Iowa, Oklahoma, North Dakota, New Hampshire, South Dakota, and Nebraska are each less than 30 percent.

While these states appear be doing very well by this indicator, it is noteworthy that Idaho recently reduced its Medicaid rates paid to nursing homes—twice—by 4 percent in July 2025, followed by another 4 percent a few months later, in September.[131]

On the other hand …

States with *highest* Debt to Asset Ratios:

- Illinois 295.58 percent
- New Jersey 249.64 percent
- New York 218.12 percent
- Connecticut 172.44 percent
- California 111.04 percent
- Hawaii 107.31 percent

What does this portend for old, sick, or old *and* sick people in these states? It is very hard to know. What is certain, however, is that this and other financial indicators predict some level of unavoidable disruption.

Why? Explaining further ...

Based on latest available data, found on www.worldpopulationreview.com, the nation's population is estimated at roughly 347 million people.

States whose debt to asset ratios are above 100 percent represent 91+ million people, or over 26 percent of the nation's population. Adding in those whose ratios are above 80 percent, and the numbers rapidly *approach 35 percent of the nation's population.*

These numbers indicate a geographic, demographic, mathematic, economic, and financial hell. Left unabated, they'll worsen.

And today they are. Among the states highlighted, Illinois, New York, California, and Hawaii have experienced negative population growth rates when calculated year-over-year, and since the 2020 COVID-19 campaign.

Based on most recent information, these states rank among the lowest nationally in interstate migration. Measured—in hours, minutes, and seconds—this is the pace at which a taxpayer is ***leaving*** these respective states:[132]

- California — 1 minute, 44 seconds
- New York — 2 minutes, 23 seconds
- Illinois — 6 minutes, 4 seconds
- Hawaii — 1 hour, 4 minutes, 14 seconds

Sooner, rather than later, governors of these states—and their voters—will be forced to choose, as corrective levers are dwindling.

The revenue side of their fiscal policy equations are risky business. Raising taxes, fees, and regulations force taxpaying individuals and businesses to evaluate the wisdom of paying more for less or moving out.

Further, states can attempt to attract businesses to their cities and towns, though those in distress are weakened compared to states—and countries—able to offer tax incentives to companies considering relocation and expansion.

Will states borrow their way out and play "kick the can"? Some will likely try. All they'll need are people and institutions to take the other side of their deals.

ᔕ

States have company in their plight. Uncle Sam is right there with them, and has admitted it.

The Social Security Administration's *Status of the Social Security and Medicare Programs—A Summary of the 2024 Annual Reports*, prepared by the Trustees of the Social Security and Medicare trust funds, including the nation's Secretaries of Treasury, Health and Human Services, Labor, and Social Security, provides details on this admission.

Details from the Summary include:[133]

Benefit	100% Payable Until	Reduced Afterward To
OASDI (Your SS check)	2033	79%
Medicare Part A	2036	89%
Medicare Parts B & D	Indefinitely	N/A

This means the Social Security and Medicare trust funds (which are distinct, not combined)—are on a major course of Ozempic, losing weight as the days, years, and eligible beneficiaries continue to advance and grow.

Soon, beneficiaries will be going on a diet, getting less in benefits and coverage—and figuring out what to do.

To learn more, look under the summary report's section, "A Message to the Public."

Quick note: This is a financial awakening. And for old, sick, or old *and* sick people, a significant disruptor. In some circles, financial modeling—accounting for future Cost of Living Adjustments (COLA)—indicates that this awakening could occur as soon as 2029 or 2030.

How'd this happen? The multiyear narrative is that these trust funds have been paying more than they've taken in. A deeper explanation is:

- Fewer taxpaying workers per eligible beneficiary
- More beneficiaries (boomers) and growing
- Decades of unrelenting healthcare inflation (per item and transaction) and overall programmatic spending

Simply put, there aren't enough Gen X, Z, and millennials to pay the freight—in a fiscal sense—to cover the geezers.

Here's the proposed solution:

" ... The Trustees recommend that lawmakers address the projected trust fund shortfalls in a timely way in order to phase in necessary changes gradually and give workers and beneficiaries time to adjust their expectations and behavior."[134]

For workers, this would mean: 1) increased payroll taxes to pump up the trust funds, and/or 2) increasing the retirement or eligibility age for a "full schedule" of benefits.

For beneficiaries, this means—in just a few years: 1) a pay cut in monthly payments, 2) means-testing for benefits, based on monthly income from other sources, or 3) changes in benefit coverage (e.g., reductions, copayments, coinsurance).

There's more: "With informed discussion, creative thinking, and timely legislative action, Social Security and Medicare can continue to protect future generations."[135]

This sentence is the essence of trustee clarity. In other words: *This isn't our problem, it's yours.*

ᏣᏕ

Painful as these facts and figures are, the impending disruption might be delayed if people could navigate everyday living while aging with independence and self-determination.

But they can't, don't want to, or maybe even *both*.

The Pew Research Center's June 2024 report, *Americans' views of government aid to poor, role in healthcare and Social Security*[136] shared these conclusions:

- 65 percent say the government has a responsibility to ensure *all* Americans have healthcare coverage.
- 79 percent say Social Security benefits shouldn't be reduced in *any* way.
- 52 percent say the government should do *more* to help the needy, even if it means going deeper into debt.

I've intentionally italicized "all," "any," and "more" to illustrate citizen, voter, taxpayer sentiment. While Pew carves up responses by political party and race, in this context, it doesn't matter. What matters is that majorities support—some by resounding margins—healthcare coverage for all, maintaining Social Security without dilution, and doing more for those who need it.

Something's gotta give. And when something does, there will be a price paid by those most affected.

Access Contraction and Market Desertion

Many, most, or all of us are unprepared for these inevitable financial disruptions. As they evolve, each will influence what, where, and how we do it.

Asked to choose, which best describes the services you receive?

Sick Care or *Health Care*

My belief? Decision-makers and people in charge are trying desperately to figure this out. While they do, the description may sort itself out organically—and locally. Maybe that's the big idea.

Let me explain. In many communities, especially small towns, histories and economies were built on a handful of durable institutions—a large employer (or two), a public school, and a general hospital. Its citizens were likely born in the town's general hospital, educated in its public school, and benefited—somehow—from the largest employer.

These institutions were relied on for generations.

In recent decades, due to population declines, tax/bond/wage/trade implications, or physical plant senescence, towns lost their largest employers, and public schools consolidated with others.

Resultingly, people drive greater distances to and from work, and put children on school buses. Life's simplicity—and their identities—are threatened.

Hospitals haven't been immunized from this disruption. Change for them—in small towns—isn't nearly over.

The Center for Healthcare Quality and Payment Reform (CHQPR), using CMS' hospital financial information, recently determined the vulnerability of rural hospitals at *immediate risk of closure*—or within two-to-three years.

Per CHQPR, "322 rural hospitals are at immediate risk of shutting down due to severe financial difficulties." States with the greatest immediate risk (by %) are headed by Connecticut (50%), Alabama (48%), Mississippi (34%) and New York (33%).[137]

Let's say these estimates are half-right. States and their small towns will be taking massive steps toward becoming *healthcare deserts*.

Yes, *deserts*.

As towns lose their hospitals, doctors, nurses, therapists, and specialists *desert* them, *leaving* massive headaches for mayors, town councils, governors, and congressional representatives in their wake.

This is profoundly impactful for small-town nursing homes. Having worked in one and overseen hundreds, rural nursing homes are incredibly dependent on hospitals in their own (or adjacent) communities.

As an administrator, I drove forty miles each way, daily, to a home in a town of 2,000 people. Closest hospitals were thirty miles away, requiring family members to make round trips when loved ones were hospitalized.

Generating patient admissions required a sixty-mile sales radius. Success depended on the home excelling at something—or many things—telling people about it, and securing trust.

One local physician serviced this community. The home's second attending physician lived in the same city as me, driving to the home almost daily.

When a hospital—the historical source of patient admissions, acute care, and part-time labor—closes, it *can* mean the end for a rural nursing home.

Census and workforce deficits add up quickly. Absent safety valves for replacements, a specialty service or market differentiator, the desert expands.

These disruptions are the industry's history. More are coming. Soon.

What This Means

Massive—and more—problems await nursing homes. Disruption is unmistakably inevitable. Big, debt-laden states. People loathing increased taxation. Social Security and Medicare trusts withering. Rural hospitals vanishing.

Which path will lawmakers, their financial modelers, and polling analysts eventually pick? We'll know soon.

Nursing homes will remain part of the nation's landscape. However, they'll play a completely different role in health—or sick—care.

The status quo will be extinguished. Homes and companies will be winners—and losers.

Creative destruction, like other industries, will be embraced. The decades-long inertia shared in previous chapters won't endure.

Pick anything, and decide if it thrived before, during, and after the pandemic—without props, PPP, or CARES Act bailouts. *And NVIDIA, the AI computing superheavyweight whose stock price increased 13X during this time, doesn't count.*

COVID, arguably, broke the world. Nursing homes weren't spared. Fragile at its core, people-reliant, technology-light, and completely dependent on public funding and sentiment ... *until the people and the sentiment ran out.*

Will people and sentiment ever return? My bet? The weak will perish, and the strong will flourish. Here's why ...

Gibbins Advisors, a healthcare restructuring advisory firm, produced this headline in its interim 2025 report on bankruptcies:[138]

"By Subsector: Senior Care and Pharma cases led volume in H1 2025 ..."

Nursing homes with weak balance sheets, limited access to capital, aging, or uncompetitive plants due to underinvestment or operating inertia, and/or landlords with limited liquidity or interest in their tenants' success could end up being occupants in this future version of hell.

Conversely, darkness isn't everywhere in the nursing home industry. Quite the contrary. There's evidence that nursing home companies and those that support them structurally and financially are doing quite well ... *thank you very much.*

Based on most recent announcements, "doing quite well" is expected to continue, delivering real damage to the narrative (or myth) that nursing homes are broken.

While nursing homes and companies have been treading water—or drowning in alleged red ink—industry heavyweight The Ensign Group is treating the industry as one big "K-Mart Blue Light Special," as illustrated in their 30 percent growth in locations since 2020:

	December 31,				
	2020[(1)]	2021[(1)]	2022[(1)]	2023[(1)]	2024
Cumulative number of skilled nursing and senior living operations	228	245	271	297	327
Cumulative number of operational skilled nursing beds	23,172	25,032	28,130	30,602	33,547
Cumulative number of senior living units	2,254	2,237	3,021	3,121	3,088

(1) Number of operational beds and number of operations for 2020-2023 include operational beds and operations that we no longer operate. The number of operations and operational beds do not include the closed facilities beginning in the year of their closures.

Source: The Ensign Group, SEC Form 10-K—2024

Buying and turning around distressed nursing homes, or homes in markets with favorable workforce availability and Medicaid payment, look like transformative opportunities for Ensign, and others following suit.

Quick note: As of 6/1/25, Ensign's cumulative number of locations was 347.

In this light, the largest disruption could occur in nursing homes and companies with deficiencies in talent, depth, capital, competence, leadership, performance, and creativity rather than the industry as a whole.

So … what is real? Behaviors of publicly held companies, in this case, Ensign—are challenging the commonly-held industrial narratives. Is this to sustain interest in their companies? Are their behaviors based on faulty intelligence, destined to fates like their peers?

I'm taking their five-year performance trend at face value, encouraged that companies are thriving within this industry.

And of the nursing homes, companies, lenders, landlords, and trade association executives painting landscapes of darkness at every turn. Are they victims of bad analytics, purveyors of chronically weak talent and balance sheets, and owners of Op and PropCos with poorly designed and executed strategies?

Or, quoting the Bee Gees—of *Saturday Night Fever* fame—are they *Jive Talkin'*?

One final disruption bears exploration, specific to people. If I were working for a nursing home company today, it would be one of my first questions:

Who requires more care—patients or caregivers?
Here's why …

- In 2021, the National Alliance on Mental Illness estimated that 57.8 million adults (22.8 percent) live with a mental illness.[139]
- In 2022, the Substance Abuse and Mental Health Services Administration estimated that 48.7 million people age 13 or older (17.3 percent) had a substance abuse disorder and 18.6 million (7.3 percent) had serious thoughts, planned, or attempted suicide in the past year.[140]
- A CDC study found that during 2021–2022, measures for 13 of 19 indicators were worse for caregivers than for noncaregivers, compared to prevalence in 2015-16, including mental distress, depression, heavy drinking, obesity, and multiple chronic conditions.[141]

Employers are foolish to ignore this multigenerational fragility affecting millions.

Chief people officers and leaders will have their hands full. Logo T-shirts, buttons, backpacks, and taglines will not satisfy these workforce realities.

Money, beyond traditional pay and benefits, will be needed. Some nursing homes and companies won't wait to address these issues. They'll create and fund effective workforce support.

AI will be a disruptive contributor that helps with this people issue. It will, however, be a while before its practical application is fully realized.

Recent search indicates Chat GPT services two and a half billion queries daily. Nursing homes and their companies are likely included in this statistic. As well they should. Generative AI—which produces text, images, video on request—eliminates and reduces operating costs.

Nursing homes have plenty of opportunities here. Marketing and promotional material. Web design. Graphics. Manuals and handbooks. Think it, and AI can do it.

Bias, and garbage in/out remain threats. Still, paying people to make flyers—for anything—is history. Instead, command an application and get out of the way.

With design and prompting, gathering and producing individual, group, team, single-site, region, or division performance metrics should be simplified.

Imagine the possibilities as barriers to performance evaluations are erased. Workers win. Bosses too. Time and attention is made available for learning and development, retaining and preparing workers for growth.

The disruption I envision evolves as providers invest in, and subsequently talk about, the benefits of AI. Some will plunge in, fully exploit use cases, and enjoy returns on their investments.

If I were operating a nursing home company today, I'd be value-engineering the savings associated with AI, and plowing additional dollars into workforce mental health and counseling programs—exceeding what any Employee Assistance Program offers—as market differentiators for people "giving it up" for their patients.

And the fate for those choosing to sit on the sidelines, waiting for groupthink from the echo chamber? *I don't know.* Either way, disruption is inevitable.

WHAT YOU CAN DO

Ask Questions About:

- Stability—financial and workforce—in rural locations
- Using AI as a difference-maker in taking care of people
- Mental health and advocacy services for patients and workers

Look for:

- Media communications regarding local nursing home and hospital closures and bankruptcies

Listen to Yourself:

- Can you see yourself or a loved one opting for cannabis or palliative care?
- How far would you drive to visit a loved one in a nursing home or hospital? Or vice versa?
- What is your Plan B if the nursing home or local hospital serving your loved one closes?

X

DISRUPTION IS HERE

At a recent conference on the future of senior living leadership, a contemporary took the podium and adjusted his glasses. His prominence was well-earned. Spanning decades, he held leadership positions in local communities, his home state, and Washington, DC.

Attendees quieted. A few found the gravitational pull of their phones irresistible. The rest were focused, like a classroom of college students attending their first lecture.

He described himself. Not as an executive or legislative influencer. As a dad and grandfather, far north of fifty—and a future consumer of care. Speaking directly to early and established career leaders—across the spectrum of senior living—and representatives from banking, medical equipment, and higher education.

Describing himself a "father of daughters," he expressed "no interest in becoming a burden, or the responsibility of his children." While he loved them and his grandchildren, having them as future caregivers was not part of his life's equation.

Then, as a future consumer—for an unknown need, time, or duration—he uttered this single sentence directly to those currently leading or supporting the vast assembly of business types serving seniors …

"Today, you don't have anything that I want to buy."

Attendees—from mid-twenties to early-sixties—didn't expect this candor. They expected another cheerleading event, or a full-on stroking to assuage their woeful plight of shortages of people and money.

Not on this day. Around the room, attendees looked chastened.

I had one reaction ... *APPLAUSE!* I felt myself smiling, laughing gently, bringing my hands together to celebrate this candid, provocative, and completely accurate viewpoint.

Why? You know.

No one wants to live (or die) in a nursing home, risking abuse, neglect, isolation, or loneliness.

No one wants to live among strangers, as frequently occurs in assisted living.

No one wants to give up their stuff, as required when downsizing to senior housing.

No one wants to see a different face daily, be disappointed when caregivers fail to show up—and when they do—be deficient in training, technique, or respect for them, their space, or belongings, each of which happens with in-home care. And ...

No one wants to "fly the white flag," surrendering to the end of their days, which is required for hospice services.

In knowing precisely *what they don't want*, people are defining *what they do want*, which, including rejecting the status quo, is tilting the age-old "silver tsunami" narrative in unanticipated directions.

This final chapter will explore the disruptions—in lifestyle, technology, and discretionary spending—responsible for this "tilt," and the present and future implications for consumers and providers alike.

Challenges to the Narrative

For over twenty-five years, keynote speakers (with many letters after their names) have told this story at nursing home and healthcare investment conferences:

"Once this tsunami of baby boomers begins, you nursing home guys are going to be in great shape for decades!"

People bought this story. Some probably still do. But they might not be looking in the right place for their market intelligence.

The demographics of boomers and their upcoming birthdays are unavoidable. It's mathematical. Books, graphs, and charts tell us so. This is where most analysts, owners, lenders, and decision-makers go for their intel.

I go somewhere else. Given my age and history, my circle is mostly contemporaries connected to nursing, nursing homes, healthcare, and the boomer and Gen X generations. This isn't what I am referring to.

Click on www.yahoo.com. There's treasure in their daily content. I go there. I dig for buried treasure.

It's in their "Comments," especially in articles about money, retirement, Medicare and Medicaid, health and life insurance, nursing homes, assisted living, elder abuse, legislation affecting seniors, and anything that is within an arm's reach of these topics. *Yahoo!* readers are bold in sharing opinions ... *on everything*. It's like gold.

Commenters are fearless in describing themselves, by age and gender, state or country, income and net worth, employment experiences, domestic situations, and other features which make it easy to gauge sentiments on issues.

Understanding that responses are flawed and the material isn't representative of any relevant statistical modeling, I use it for what's at its core ... *emotion*. Raw, richly unedited, and real emotion.

And what these emotional, personal, and deep responses indicate is: "Today, you don't have anything that I want to buy."

Having reviewed daily responses—for years—there has been no reversal in sentiment.

Instead of charts, surveys and traditional intel-gathering approaches, keynote speakers might invest a few hundred hours a year scoping *Yahoo! Comments* to see how they stack up with their material.

Just saying.

People Love Their Homes and Families

One disruptor—now, and in years ahead—finds families *rewinding their clocks* in their living arrangements.

Prior to living in a trailer park and moving into the rented, single-family home in which I grew up, my brothers and I spent a few years living with my parents in the home owned by my grandparents ... *with my grandparents*. Three generations under one roof.

This was quite common in early 1960s northeastern Pennsylvania.

Intergenerational living has always been a thing. I believe it will become even bigger.

During the Great Financial Crisis of 2008–09, and for years afterward, the narrative was that recent college graduates, student-debt laden, seeking work or unable to afford a mortgage, sought refuge with their parents, gaining the financial wherewithal *to move out and get a move on.*

In the mid-2020s, the narrative is similar ... but different.

Certainly, the barrier-driven dynamic involving young people, college debt, weak credit, and pay inequity continues. Parents have adjusted to this, during and post-COVID, expanding their homes to accommodate *tenant children* until market forces correct for the undersupply of new housing starts and mortgage interest rates not experienced in generations.

Today, the math on selling homes ... *sucks*. Interest rates are no longer near zero. Home prices are downright shocking. "Rate-locked" homeowners with mortgage interest rates of 2, 3, or 4 percent are reluctant to sell, even at premium prices, as their next residence will likely come with an interest rate double or triple what they've grown used to.

I remember 14, 15, 16 percent mortgages, and bought homes at these rates, when they were worth buying. Like most things, they weren't forever. Other boomers share this history, as have members of the Silent Generation.

That is where this experiential train *stops*. Will it ever restart in the US?

I wouldn't dare forecast what mortgage rates will ultimately normalize to, though I will take a leap and bet that decades of zero-interest or low, low single-digit rates are gone.

What does any of this have to do with the future of nursing homes? I believe that it has the potential, like Ozempic, Wegovy, and Mounjaro, to put a severe hurting on the demand for nursing home services.

Why? No one wants to live in a nursing home, and people will do anything possible to stay out of a nursing home.

I'm seeing this behavior today, up-close and personal, and at a distance. People are *rewinding their clocks*, using traditional and creative approaches.

How? Here are a few examples:

- Boomers are requesting, and receiving zoning approval to site a prefabricated small home on single-family home parcels, serving as a "mother-in-law's" quarters, and an alternative to assisted living, continuing care retirement communities, or skilled nursing. In these situations, zoning approval is contingent, and limited to applicant-only occupation. Others are converting (or constructing) space to apartments, renting space through Airbnb until parents or in-laws are ready to occupy.
- Adult children are moving in with elderly boomers and members of the Silent Generation, supporting and caring for their parents as an alternative to institutional care, and concurrently mitigating risks associated with asset liquidation (and estate degradation) and incidents that would result in admission to a more restrictive setting.
- Boomers (and elders) and their children are executing sale-and-leaseback arrangements where the parents remain in the home as tenants and adult children are landlords. Proceeds from these transactions can help underwrite in-home equipment, adaptations, and services, or to spend—rather than pursue reverse mortgage arrangements with financial institutions. In

> some situations, adult children move in, supporting their parents with activities of daily living, and forgoing the need for institutional care.

This is what people *are doing* to stay at home, and near their families.

ꟹ

Understandably, skeptics will dismiss anecdotes in favor of narratives which suit them. It's what people do. When big business gets involved in a movement, however, skeptics are wise to take notice. Let me explain ...

Lennar Homes's *Next Gen* home, promoted as, "The Home Within a Home," is "designed to accommodate two homes under one roof, perfect for aging parents, adult children or extended family members. [It] allows for a harmonious living where everyone has their own space—all while still being part of the family."[142]

If you're unfamiliar with Lennar Corporation, they are a homebuilding *giant*, with reported 2024 gross revenues of $35+ billion.[143] For a big public company, they must see a compelling business reason to provide this offering to people interested in new home construction.

I think Lennar sees a trend—a big, growing one. Not a fad.

I also think Lennar, and others, see the opportunity in giving families *solutions*. Solutions to what's impeded young people for parts of the last fifteen years, and fears and anxieties which prospective nursing home patients and their loved ones have grappled with for seven decades.

A tagline for Lennar's NextGen could have been, "Let us build you a house that takes care of everyone."

If I were the adult child of a parent living in a rural community who might need skilled nursing someday, and local nursing home providers were lamenting their future prospects—including diminished access to care—any, *or all*, of these options would be fodder for discussion and planning.

Hospitals Love Keeping People in Their Homes

Everyday people aren't the only ones rejecting the status quo. Quietly, beginning in the 1990s, thought leaders from Johns Hopkins University School of Medicine and The John A. Hartford Foundation began reimagining acute care—providing it in one's home.

This disruptor, called Hospital-at-Home (H@H), is exactly that. Neither Hopkins nor The Hartford Foundation minces words on this, as evidenced by these statements:

"Hospital care is not ideal for many older patients."[144]

"Hospitals are without a doubt the most expensive and dangerous places to receive your healthcare. They are particularly unsafe for older adults, who experience a disproportionate burden of complications, functional decline, harm, and even death as inpatients."[145]

You know. Disorientation, infection, injury or illness, a material change in condition, fear, loneliness, and more.

From The American Hospital Association, this is "How It Works":[146]

- Patients are determined as program-eligible when they're seen in a hospital emergency department or ambulatory care center.
- If eligible, patients aren't admitted. Instead, they return home for care and treatment.
- Nurses address patient needs at least daily, or more frequently as assessed.
- Physicians use a combination of telemedicine and in-person house calls to see their patients at least once daily.
- Nurses and physicians are available 24/7 for urgent issues.
- Diagnostic studies and therapeutic treatments occur at home.
- When medically stable, the patient is discharged from the program.

Prime candidates for this program include those with pneumonia, congestive heart failure, COPD (or emphysema), cellulitis, dehydration, urinary tract infections, and deep vein thrombosis (DVT) among others. Or conditions customarily attributed to people admitted to nursing homes following hospitalization.

Nearing its thirtieth anniversary, this concept has survived testing. A 2024 CMS study indicated, when compared to bricks and mortar hospitals, H@H patients experienced decreased mortality, lower Medicare spending in the thirty days post-discharge, and predominantly positive views among patients and caregivers.[147]

This has been cause for applause. Over time, results have attracted attention, support, and money.

In 2015, with CMS grant funding, the Icahn School of Medicine at New York's Mount Sinai began testing the creation of a Medicare payment model, with further study funded by The Hartford Foundation.

This movement caught fire during, and since, COVID.

- In April 2021, CMS reported 127 participating hospitals in twenty-nine states.[148]
- In September 2024, CMS reported 332 participating hospitals in thirty-eight states.[149]
- As of July 2025, The American Hospital Association reported 400 participating hospitals in thirty-nine states.[150]

This is what momentum and rejection of the status quo looks like. Sorting through names of participating health systems, it's easy to forecast where this program could be going. Here's a brief sampling

Mount Sinai

Mass General Brigham

University of Utah Huntsman Cancer Institute

Intermountain Health System

Presbyterian Healthcare Services

Marshfield Medical Centers

Mayo Clinic

Cleveland Clinic

Geisinger Health

Kaiser Permanente

Baylor Scott & White Health

Medical University of South Carolina

University of Florida

Orlando Health

Beth Israel Deaconess Lahey Health

These, and other acute care heavyweights, indicate a commitment where disruption is near guaranteed. The lone barrier to guaranteed expansion is the tenuous state of the program—extended by congressional waiver, through 2030.

This extension likely means more hospitals offering this service in communities, adding disruption to those nursing homes whose business model is built on high volumes and turnover of short-stay patients.

In the continually developing world of value-based care and bundled payments, hospitals can, should, and will take control of what's within reach, eliminating or reducing reliance on nursing homes, and providing care where patients want it—*in their homes.*

Other hospitals and health systems, rather than flying solo, choose joint venture (JV) partners—like Contessa Health—to execute their H@H strategies.

Through contracts with insurance companies or their JV partners, Contessa assumes limited or full financial risk for cost-effectively coordinating care in the home. In addition to their H@H capabilities, they also offer a skilled nursing facility at-home (SNF@H) option to payors, providers, and their clients.

There are big-league players, as illustrated by the names found at www.contessahealth.com:

Henry Ford Health

Highmark Health

Marshfield Clinic Health System

Mount Sinai

Penn State Health

University of Arkansas for Medical Sciences (UAMS)

They appear to be good at it too. In June 2021, home care and hospice provider Amedisys (NASDAQ:AMED) purchased Contessa for *$250 million.*[151]

No bricks and mortar. Just talented people with a way to give people what they want.

Two years later, Optum, a business owned by UnitedHealth Group (NYSE:UNH), offered to buy Amedisys for north of *$3 billion.*[152] This move occurred *less than six months after* Optum finalized the acquisition of an Amedisys competitor, LHC Group—for *$5.4 billion.*[153]

With an approved deal in hand, and working through Department of Justice and Federal Trade Commission requirements, Optum and Amedisys's market moves—involving billions—signifies that Hospital @ Home, and other things being "Done @ Home" isn't going away.

What this means for nursing homes, historically reliant on health systems and their hospitals for patient referrals, is that they'll need to earn—and keep—a seat at the table among payors, health systems, their hospitals, and JV partners.

This will be neither easy nor fun.

Winners will be forced to invest in their assets—people, plant, and process—delivering outcomes that fit what their payors and partners demand. Efficient, compliant, well-governed, and capitalized nursing homes and companies have big days ahead.

Those challenged in these areas will eventually be boxed out, forced into change, wrestling with survival.

In either case, they'll wave goodbye to formerly prospective patients as they receive hospital services—*at home.*

ယ

If the thesis of *home* increasingly becoming the locus of healthcare has appeal, this anecdote may pique your interest. Not long ago, my wife and I participated in a webinar on an investment opportunity—with a few twists.

Sponsors were people we'd done business with for years, who were now reflecting on lifestyle opportunities for long-term business partners. Most participants were far north of the *Big 5-oh*, working to squeeze every remaining ounce of life on the one hand—and preparing for when it ended, on the other.

Midway through, the conversation pivoted from the investment's value proposition and short-term goals to longer-term ambitions, including the creation of living communities for members.

Intentionally avoiding specifics, the tone was different yet inspiring. It didn't involve a traditional product or service, like a continuing care retirement community (CCRC) or assisted living offering. Or a Del Webb-type arrangement, where builders and buyers operate in distinct lanes, strangers are many, homeowner association (HOA) fees and assessments bring surprises, and experiences are unpredictable.

Instead, this encompassed building a neighborhood of people with common interests and experiences, who would assemble, pull together, and take care of each other as they ran, walked, shuffled, or rolled down the back stretch of life.

It would include a medical feature, where doctors in concierge practices made house calls, a relationship with an accredited hospital providing advanced-level in-home services, and—where necessary—the mutual underwriting of care needed and provided.

The architecture and execution of this latter point would be fully dependent on whether this community resided in the US or involved senior medical tourism in a foreign land. Building upon the premise that people don't sue their friends—medical malpractice and patient liability challenges would be given no quarter.

In any case, this idea was built on self-determination and independence—which we've explored and will further.

Rewinding the clock, indeed.

Big Tech, Big Opportunities

Curbside delivery has been a massive post-COVID disruptor. Major companies have redesigned their core business strategies around it. Some successfully. Others—not even close.

As consumers, you know the companies and what works or doesn't.

Telemedicine was another disruptor that emerged into broad-based consumer consciousness. Love it or leave it, visual access to a doctor or nurse was a worthwhile alternative to risking already compromised health—by camping in the nation's waiting rooms and emergency departments.

Contemporary living is unimaginable without these two *former* disruptors, at least until they're replaced with something different and better. That might be on the way.

I'll use curbside delivery at places like Home Depot and Lowe's, especially for items too awkward or heavy to deadlift into my car.

As this feature lives on in retail, Amazon and others continue door-to-door, same day, and next-day service. This is unbeatable—for many things.

It does, however, have risks. Drivers mixing up delivery addresses. Fumbles and drops resulting in material and product damage. Leaving heavy boxes at the bottom, rather than the tops, of stairs. Add porch-pirating to these headaches and the luster of home delivery suffers intermittent tarnishing.

Amazon, knowing this for some time, has another disruptor waiting patiently. Here's a headline from their website:

"Amazon's drones deliver items in sixty minutes or less—here's how we simplified the process."

A May 2024, AP News article "Amazon gets FAA approval allowing it to expand drone deliveries for online orders," reported the company received approval to provide drone-based delivery service "beyond the visual line of sight," removing a "barrier that has prevented drones from traveling longer distances."[154]

This allowed Amazon to advance testing—initiated in College Station, Texas, market, late-2022—and its strategy to deliver online orders via drones, something that the company has discussed publicly for years.

Until then, Amazon—and Wal-Mart—required human spotters for its drone delivery research and development. This safety requirement made this undertaking expensive, limiting scalability and profitability.

With this now history, Amazon, through its Prime Air program, and Wal-Mart, testing in the Dallas-Fort Worth market, will establish and sustain momentum in the 'burbs, and out in the country. In Wal-Mart's case, I typed in "Wal-Mart drone delivery," finding everything needed about how the program works and what's eligible for delivery.

Through the FAQs, I learned that "there is no order minimum" and "there is no cost for drone delivery at this time."

This disruptor is here to stay. It'll get bigger too.

People away from the fray who can't drive, ride, or shop yet can get a friend or neighbor to catch and fetch their food items, toilet paper—and even medications—stand a fighting chance of maintaining their independence and preserving their right of self-determination.

ᔕᔓ

Ever hear of LiDAR, or Waymo? No, these are not punk rock bands from the 1980s, though if this were your guess, it would not be laughed off by good friends. In time, these terms might become as familiar as antilock brakes did in the 1990s, or Garmin in the 2000s.

LiDAR, or light detection and ranging, uses sensors to help computerized systems identify things—people, animals, and obstacles—in a real-life environment, for example, when driving down a road or highway.

Waymo is a division of Alphabet (Google), whose core business involves the creation and adoption of autonomous or self-driving ride hailing services. Yes. Big words and Buck Rogers-type stuff. One sentence explains this:

Waymo is Uber or Lyft, but without a driver.

Relying on LiDAR, and every available upgrade, Waymo gives people rides, in cars, by themselves, safely, every day. They have a program called Waymo One, which can be downloaded on the Apple App Store, or secured via Google Pay.

And they're road bound, serving Phoenix, San Francisco, LA, Atlanta, and Austin markets, with more markets to come—Vegas, San Diego, Washington DC, Denver, and Miami. Why? Because Google, I mean Alphabet, is a company proven to have the ability to tilt the world and doesn't do things simply for exercise.

For years, I've been a Google shareholder and a spectator of what they do. I think they will do *way mo' with Waymo*.

What's this have to do with independence and self-determination? *Everything*. Paratransit services will change. People will call or log on to Waymo or a competing service, like they do today, hail a car, go *wherever*, and return.

Calls to adult children, neighbors, and friends seeking rides to *wherever* will end—unless the person seeking a ride wants company—or needs help transferring in and out of the car.

People with an entrepreneurial twist will decide to buy one (or more) of these autonomous vehicles, become a "car-lord," and make these cars available to the market, doing the same thing that Uber, Lyft, Waymo, and Bob's Your Uncle transportation service does—give people rides.

This disruptor will keep people in their own homes longer, providing the flexibility and freedom missing today in getting from Point A to Point B, without risk, drama, or a lecture from adult children.

Eventually, their adult children will do Waymo too.

ᔕ

Drones aren't the only air-bound disruptors on our horizons. If a car, drone, and helicopter had a child (use your imagination, please), you might end up with this next disruptor.

Say hello to eVTOL, or electric vertical take-off and landing aircraft. It's exactly as named. It goes up in the air, then comes down.

I learned about these creations and their companies, like Joby Aviation and Archer Aviation, at a multiday investor conference designed to present new ideas to people interested in new ideas.

And this was new. Before seeing live footage, I envisioned helicopters. Interesting and ballsy, though not new. I've done some helicopter travel and have great appreciation for the use cases, piloting talent, and agility. I also appreciated two other features of this travel—*noise and price.*

Presenters played their video. It was like watching an episode of *The Jetsons*. In congested areas, like big cities, these things would become massive difference-makers.

Barriers to independence or self-determination, like sitting in a Waymo for an hour and needing to pee, or time delays due to jammed traffic ... gone with eVTOL.

City dwellers—and someday, probably suburbanites—can go down the elevator of their high-rise, take Waymo to Signature Aviation or a participating luxury hotel with a helipad, and use their app to take a ride beneath the clouds to see a friend, get to an appointment or an airport where a valet provides escort service to their airline check-in, gate, and seat.

eVTOL manufacturers tout a range of 100 miles, with speeds between 150–200 miles per hour, and seating for up to four passengers. To achieve scale, these service providers will have to compete with taxi providers. Time will tell us whether this is possible.

Time will also tell us if their drone-like features can be fully exploited, resulting in autonomous flight.

Instead of "Look Mom, no hands!" it would be "Look Mom, no pilot!"

You can picture this. Ending the agony of big city traffic, shitty parking options, angry and distracted drivers routinely blowing red lights, makes this disruptor an attention-getter.

As a veteran of subway and commuter trains, I've seen enough rats the size of dogs, watched enough people relieve themselves on platforms, and witnessed enough hand-to-hand and domestic violence for a lifetime.

Yeah ... for the right price and eardrum preservation, I'd look seriously at taking a George Jetson-ride when my thirst for battles on the asphalt—or in the tunnels—wanes.

And if the alternative is sitting on my ass in an assisted living facility or nursing home, simply because I can no longer get from where I am to where I want to be ... I'd be downloading the app and learning where and when these flying cars leave and return—today—for as long as I could.

☙

One final technology-based disruptor might evoke instant smirks or *calling BS* for stretching beyond conventional limits. Nevertheless, this opportunity has industrial momentum, gargantuan money behind it, and use cases galore.

If you remember the characters from the *Star Wars* franchise, or Rosie from *The Jetsons*, you know where this leads. Robotics—or more specifically, autonomous humanoid robots.

OK ... let me explain.

Years ago, my attention expanded to include Elon Musk. Frankly, it couldn't be avoided. The guy is everywhere. The only place he isn't—at least in person—is sitting at our kitchen table.

And he says things that leave impressions. Love him or not, you have to give him that.

When Musk and Tesla began sharing thoughts about its Optimus robot, I began digging through articles and links. Same for Boston Dynamics and their Atlas version, for reasons related to solving nursing home workforce problems and the possibilities for everyday people at home.

I figured ... why not? Businesses have been using them, whole or in part, for decades. With safety and dexterity, robotics has great utility as a workforce supplement.

Consider this—something that requires only a charged battery and preventive maintenance, can work three shifts, with no call-ins, no workers' comp, or bolting to the competition for an extra twenty-five cents an hour.

The alternatives?

- Having no one to do the work
- Grinding workers to nothingness with extra shifts and overtime
- Deploying relative strangers from a temporary staffing agency

The possibilities can't be ignored.

Visit YouTube or search *robotics* and *workplace*, and let it rip. Fascinating things are happening, ranging from the precise and delicate to hard things that not enough people want to do.

Companies can rent robots today—for the day, week, or month. Prices I've seen advertised range from $10/day and up. I've heard talking heads toss out purchase prices of $20,000 to $50,000/robot.

Generally speaking, at these prices or even higher, this movement is not outlandish to imagine. I base this on visible, daily consumer behavior.

People *will* pay $50,000 (and more) for a Ford F-150, leaving it parked and unused for twenty-to-twenty-three hours a day. They'll do the same with a luxury car and pay twice that.

And during mass production, these *devices*—motorized vehicles—include many tasks performed exclusively through robotics. Assembly, welding, painting, and quality control of every vehicle probably traces back to a robot—or a robotic something.

If I really needed one someday, I'd buy a robot. I probably wouldn't be driving (thanks eVTOL or Waymo), and wouldn't be thrilled about a live-in, nonfamily member caregiver. When the time came, this option would probably be smarter, cheaper, and maybe even better.

Why not?

Hey, if Alexa can shuffle songs and find me everything from the '70s, I'm willing to bet that someday Al, Albert, or Alicia might be able to bring me a sliced kielbasa "sanguich" with sauerkraut and hot mustard, along with an iced tea and the clicker when I rotate from the bedroom or bathroom to my favorite chair to watch the game.

If I needed an assist from my seat-lift chair, Albert could help wrap a gait belt around—or hand me my walker—making sure that I got to bed safe and in one piece, before I plugged him in next to my phone, iPad, and whatever code or panic alert system is the standard.

If my vitals—detected by a wearable ring or wristband—go sideways, Albert, linked to the device that measures and records my vitals, awakens and pushes this information directly to the 24/7 RN care manager, courtesy of a developing partnership today between NVIDIA and start-up company Hippocratic AI, who I pay $39.95 monthly to maintain a constant, but distant, eye on me, answering questions and providing expert advice.

Should my vitals threaten my continued existence—or I fall down and can't get up—Albert, via direct 10G connectivity (or whatever's in place by then), hails a subscription-based, driverless, concierge EMS—*where the paramedics are totally devoted to me*—and meets them at my front door upon arrival, as this is an added feature of my monthly program.

Long before Al moves in to be my valet/cook/aide/home secretary, I'll wholeheartedly support a tax credit for people or families that buy their own autonomous humanoid robot. It's far cheaper than the state paying for a patient's nursing home stay under Medicaid, replaces general and professional liability disputes with product litigation, and is one person less for the existing, stretched regulatory system to be responsible for oversight.

Think this is outlandish or even … stupid? *Maybe.* If not, what a disruptor it would be, yes? It would revolutionize how people could extend their independence while maintaining their ability to self-determine.

Amazingly, twenty-five or thirty years ago, people said the internet was a passing fad, rhetorically critical of its boundless possibilities. It was considered a time-waster, an on-ramp for gaming or a vehicle for doing things for entertainment's sake. A question for the naysayers: *How'd that work out?*

Let's go back to the article "The Internet? Bah!," found in the February 27, 1995 issue of *Newsweek*, written by its technology expert and columnist Clifford Stoll, in which he told readers, "… cyberspace isn't, and will never be, nirvana."[155]

This prediction became unforgettable.

Stoll will be remembered for his *1995* prediction that *the internet would be toast by … 1996.*

Among his many "truths," these might be his most regrettable:

"The truth is no online database will replace your daily newspaper, no CD-ROM can take the place of a competent teacher and no computer network will change the way the government works."[156]

I've read interviews and articles about Stoll's prognostications, and it seems like he has survived 1995 with grace. Good for him. Being wrong sucks, and it hurts. He was, however, undeniably right about the irreplaceability of a great teacher. Still, massive props to Clifford Stoll for putting it out there in the first place.

Last Calls

These final chapters provided a mix of topics worthy of optimism and dread. Certain developments will become reality in our lifetimes, while others will emerge during the lives of our children and grandchildren. Others won't materialize, and for those ideas I simply will be ... *wrong.*

That's OK. Better to go to bat and strike out than sit in dugout and not take the field, or worse—sit in the stands and watch.

Wrapping up thoughts on medical momentum, lifestyle demands, increasing desire for self-determination, and financial realities and awakenings, I'll make a good faith attempt to incorporate this work with one person's imagination of future possibilities.

So, here we go ...

It's not hard to imagine an environment where GLP-1 agonists like Ozempic, Wegovy, and Mounjaro help people improve and extend their lives, reefer is recognized for its medicinal purposes, and answers are found to stop—or slow down—the heartbreak of Alzheimer's, Parkinson's, and other diseases. Any combination of these developments results in massive, beneficial disruptions for people whose lives are shorter, or harder, than they would like.

It's not hard to rewind the clock and imagine multiple generations living under one roof, or on a common acreage footprint, strengthening bonds and memories, making the most of what time, money, and togetherness provides. As they become sick, people are treated through the computer, by brilliant people with skilled hands and big hearts, who might appear in person—in their own living rooms—rather than suffering the avoidable and intolerable experiences associated with in-patient hospitalization.

It's not hard to imagine like-minded people, buying or building their own life communities, with the goal of being with and around those they love—and making them feel good—until their life's clock hits 0:00, rather than continually negotiating barriers to things they enjoy.

It's not hard to imagine science creating a personal living environment where driverless cars and planes replace the challenge and risk of travel, blasting gaping holes through the real-life threats of isolation and loneliness, or having your own robotic maid, butler, valet, or personal assistant, connected to first responders, health professionals, and one's own personal network—all day, every day.

It's not hard to imagine a shift toward respect and dignity for those in pain—acute of heart, or chronic of body—where the senses of sight, smell, touch, and listening are valued beyond their intrinsic nature, and professionals and practitioners of these specialties are recognized and rewarded for their personal, educational, and experiential investments in providing comfort to others.

On the other hand ...

It's almost impossible to imagine a day when the nation's elected and appointed officials and voting and non-voting public ultimately agree on matters involving money, people, and taking care of one another. Specific to healthcare, many will work to support the industry, using the federal government as their bogeyman, through Federal Financial Participation, Provider Tax, and Intergovernmental Transfer payment programs as often as allowed.

It's not hard, however, to imagine a day when the nation's governors will be forced to change. In a macro sense, everything about everything is a numbers game, and a day will come when the numbers become too big to continue the *same ol' same ol'*.

It's not hard to imagine a day when leadership emerges—within states or a group of states—and promises and platforms are kept, helping those most in need, supporting the disenfranchised, rooting out the fraudsters, charlatans, and BS artists that take and don't give back, applying the principle of "First, Do No Harm" on behalf of their constituents. And ...

It's not hard to imagine a day when people, even though *they may not want to*, reject the status quo, invest in themselves and the life given to them, and pull on every available string to maintain their independence, determining what's best for them—for as long as they can.

Add to this imaginative exercise White House support for home and community-based services, an evolving expectation of hospitals as the nation's gatekeepers of health (or sick) care, and the increasing root structure of Medicare Advantage and Medicaid Managed Care giants like Centene, Elevance (formerly Anthem), Molina, Aetna/CVS, and UnitedHealth Group. The threats to the nation's nursing homes are real.

Their role in our nation's future landscape remains unwritten. Economists, bankers, lenders, and opinion-makers predict their boon is rapidly approaching. My belief, shared throughout these chapters, is it will be hard for nursing homes to serve—futuristically—at levels equal to or greater than its present or past.

Given the shifting landscape, those that endure will have to be incredibly strong in all features of patient care, people management, and business results to be invited to *any* reindeer games.

ᔓ

Again, it's hard to imagine a nation without nursing homes. It's not hard to imagine something completely disrupted in health (or sick) care where nursing homes are concerned.

Lessons learned from the industry's historical fragmentation and recent performance, it's easy to believe that as nursing homes are "retired" due to senescence, and funding, financing, and satisfying consumer (taxpayer/voter) sentiment further evolves, they will play a more specialized—and reduced—role in the person-centered life experience.

Where real money is involved, hospitals will rely on nursing homes able to achieve a distinct mission. For people unable to be cared for through a Hospital-at-Home program, metropolitan-area nursing homes with strong, stable affiliations and demonstrable histories of providing excellent care to people with complex needs will be leaned on heavily.

Hospital-like in service delivery, these homes will provide a lower cost alternative for those "holding the bag of money," preparing short-term patients for next steps in their life's journey better, faster, and cheaper than historical competitors—or the hospitals themselves. They may be designated, and paid, differently than today, which could be a very good thing.

Other homes, specializing in memory care, behavior management, or substance use disorders, will serve a community need based on services provided and full participation in state Medicaid programs. Financial survival will depend on the formulas supporting these living environments, with features that may look something like those in place today—*or completely different.*

Municipalities, responding to taxpayer/voter sentiment—may rewind their own clocks—subsidizing or outright owning homes in counties or towns, caring for those in need. Historically, these investments ended up becoming painful line items of city, town, and county budgets, drawing the ire of taxpayers or newly arriving resident/taxpayer/voters, and *eventually* becoming recycled as a community center, or torn down for a softball/baseball complex. Nevertheless, the potentiality of healthcare desertion in rural communities will restore this agenda item among town councils.

Today, homes that are neither specialized, nor special, are destined to become casualties once disruption reaches its peak. Weak capital structures, uninventive leadership, and thought leaders clinging to a belief that all homes should be winners will likely be disappointed.

Like today in other business sectors, and since the creation of the Medicare and Medicaid Act of 1965, these homes will become candidates for the Polsinelli-TrBK indices, eventually finding themselves in Chapter 11, later purchased at "blue light special" prices per bed and resuscitated by companies that are good at, and like being, in the nursing home business—or by companies in other industries that turn this valuable real estate into something completely different.

And when this happens, this will be a good thing.

It's with these ideas in mind that it's hard to imagine a nation without nursing homes. There will always be a need for places to care for people who are unable to take care of themselves.

ꕥ

Unlike other chapters, this one doesn't end with a series of prompts to "Ask, Look, and Listen." If you've come this far, you don't need it.

With what you've learned, and what you know, you're prepared to critically examine a multitude of items on a critically complex, important matter—taking the best care of yourself or a loved one.

The "Myths and Truths," as shared in these chapters, are unknown to a disproportionate share of people residing, visiting, working, supporting, and overseeing nursing homes today.

But not to you.

Navigate confidently. Share your knowledge with others. Remain curious.

ACKNOWLEDGMENTS

Bringing an idea—this book—to life, was daunting and at times humbling. Much like building a house, converting a vision to a reality requires help across a spectrum of areas.

Through the leadership and experience Amanda Miller and My Word Publishing brought to the project, the unfamiliar became relatable, the complex simplified, and the scary—wasn't. Thanks for helping me realize that "I'm a Writer." And, it very much is a superpower. And additional thanks for introducing me to your network of world-class experts, the likes of which I'd never met, came to know, and learned from working with.

Words assembled in sentences lack meaning and impact without structure and sequence. Expert coaching and guidance from Laura Kaiser and Word Haven Editorial resulted in "honing" for conciseness while retaining and clarifying meaningful thoughts, insights, and opinions. Thank you, Laura, for challenging the entirety of this work—from first to final word.

Thanks also to Cheryl Jaclin Isaac for polishing this work delivered to you in its final form. Proofreading is exacting and essential, and it's been my great fortune to benefit from Cheryl's fine work.

Award-winning designer Laura Duffy expertly shaped this book's cover, creating its visual identity and helping it to stand out in a crowded, competitive landscape, while Asya Blue delivered equal beauty in layout and interior pages formatting. Thank you both for your creativity and artistry.

Last, thanks to the entire team at Layton Road Press, for tying off the remaining loose ends behind this work.

Many friends and colleagues reviewed multiple drafts, providing valuable commentary on tone and content. Thank you Amita Avadhani, Tony and Patrice Baker, Steve Brigance, Brian Bursa, Dona Carpenter, Jenn Ibrahim, Elaine Johnston, Keith Knapp, Steve Kisty, Suzy Kraky, John Kranick, Andy Kush, Doug Olson, Paul Porvaznik, Scott Sidman, Lisa Thomson, Kirsten Ullman, and Debi Witt.

Special thanks to Ralph Datto, David Mills, and Karen Vincent, each of whom read every version produced over a three-year stretch, sharing their insights and encouragement, and repeatedly replying, "Send more." Your confidence in me and courage to share—even when the feedback was unpopular—was invaluable.

Thanks also to my interested crewmates from the Northeast Georgia Officials Association, for their support and encouragement in continuing this work during the 2023 and 2024 football seasons. Many pre-game and halftime conversations included, "How's the Book?" and "When will it be done?"

Once initiated, this project dominated my daily attention, across continents. During visits to South Africa (twice), Nicaragua (thrice), and Portugal, the laptop was open for additions and revisions, between game drives to seek Cape Buffalo or kudu, before watching Pacific sunsets, or walking thousands (and thousands) of steps in the Algarve. A massive thank you to Melissa Karron, our team captain at Africa Through Your Lens, in finding me time, space, and electricity when it was in short supply.

I'd be remiss in not recognizing two people who profoundly impacted my respect for the written word, and the desire to pursue this project—the late Carol Datto, who taught me the importance of applying deep thought to the reading experience, and John Hockin, who inspired young readers to take risks and write stories of their own. Though their guidance is nearly fifty years old, it lives on in this work.

Mom's passing halfway through this experience forced me to examine myself and everything that mattered. While many things endured—or didn't—devotion to this work strengthened. Thank you, Ann Davis, forever. For everything. My one wish is that you were able to have turned through these pages. I think you'd have liked it.

A heartfelt thank you to my daughters—Christine, Mary, and Andrea—each of whom routinely asked for progress updates and supported the risks taken in sharing stories and baring opinions. Additionally, thank you for your understanding and love across the decades when work took me away from home, many times for extended periods and at the expense of attending your games, concerts, assemblies, and other events. As I've said and often wrote, being your dad is the best job I'll ever have.

Ideas often result in interesting, though empty, conversations. In the early 2010s, the idea for this work followed completing a grueling expert witness engagement, followed days later by the initial draft of this book's preface. Ten years later, I revisited this idea with my love, partner, friend, and biggest fan, who encouraged me to share every thought of consequence, inform and educate at every opportunity, ignore the slings and arrows of likely critics, and deliver work that engaged and entertained readers. Thank you, Patrice, for the support and encouragement—over nearly twenty-five years—that made considering and executing this work possible. I do love you so.

ENDNOTES

Chapter I: Many People Are Afraid of Nursing Homes

1 Priya Chidambaram and Alice Burns, "A Look at Nursing Facility Characteristics in 2025," *Kaiser Family Foundation*, December 17, 2025, https://www.kff.org/medicaid/a-look-at-nursing-facility-characteristics/.

2 https://www.quotetab.com/quote/by-bette-davis/getting-old-isnt-for-sissies.

3 Atul Gawande, "Being Mortal – Medicine and What Matters in the End," *Metropolitan Books/Henry Holt and Company*, 2014, https://atulgawande.com/book/being-mortal/.

Chapter II: The Disrespect for Nursing Home Patients Is an Open Secret

4 Phyllis Shelton, "What your state lets you keep, effective 7/1/2025," *The ABC's of Long Term Care Insurance,* July 1, 2025, https://gotltci.com/2025/01/what-your-state-lets-you-keep.

5 "How Much Monthly Income Can be Kept When Residing in a Medicaid-Funded Nursing Home?," *American Council on Aging*, July 28, 2025, https://www.medicaidplanningassistance.org/personal-needs-allowance.

6 John Waggoner and Andy Markowitz, "History of Social Security COLA Increases by Year", *AARP,* Published July 16, 2021,Updated October 10, 2024 https://www.aarp.org/social-security/cola-history/.

7 "Can Money Buy You Happiness?," *Fantastic Facts,* https://fantasticfacts.net/6252.

8 "Gertrude Stein Quotes", *Brainy Quote,* https://www.brainyquote.com/quotes/gertrude_stein_163501.

9 "AHCA/NCAL President Mark Parkinson Talks Long Term Care Efforts to Battle Spread of Coronavirus," *YouTube*, March 10, 2020, https://www.youtube.com/watch?v=7TKllyd92Is.

10 Joshua Montes, Christopher Smith, and Juliana Dajon, ""The Great Retirement Boom": The Pandemic-Era Surge in Retirements and Implications for Future Labor Force Participation," *Board of Governors of the Federal Reserve System*, November 2022, https://www.federalreserve.gov/econres/feds/the-great-retirement-boom.htm.

11 "REPORT: Nursing Homes Down 221,000 Jobs Since Start of Pandemic," *AHCA/NCAL*, November 10, 2021, https://www.ahcancal.org/News-and-Communications/Press-Releases/Pages/REPORT-Nursing-Homes-Down-221,000-Jobs-Since-Start-Of-Pandemic.aspx.

12 Alex Zorn, "No Magic Bullet: How "No Magic Bullet: How Operators are Rethinking Their Staffing Strategies", *Skilled Nursing News,* May 25, 2022, https://skillednursingnews.com/2022/05/no-magic-bullet-how-operators-are-rethinking-their-staffing-strategies.

13 "Long Term Care Jobs Report", *AHCA/NCAL,* January 2023, https://www.ahcancal.org/News-and-Communications/Fact-Sheets/FactSheets/LTC-Jobs-Report-Jan2023.pdf.

14 Tim Mullaney, "Strained by Survey Challenges, Nursing Home Operators Cite Inexperienced Inspection Teams," *Skilled Nursing News*, July 23, 2023, https://skillednursingnews.com/2023/07/strained-by-survey-challenges-nursing-home-operators-cite-inexperienced-inspection-teams.

15 Amy Stulick, "Staffing Shortages Cause Survey Backlog for Half of Connecticut SNFs, in Tandem With More Immediate Jeopardy Cases," *Skilled Nursing News*, July 31, 2023, https://staging.skillednursingnews.com/2023/07/staffing-shortages-cause-survey-backlog-for-half-of-connecticut-snfs-in-tandem-with-more-immediate-jeopardy-cases.

16 U.S. Senate Special Committee on Aging, "Uninspected & Neglected - Final Report," March 21, 2024, https://www.documentcloud.org/documents/24491852-us-senate-special-committee-on-aging-uninspected-neglected-final-report.

17 Ibid.

18 Rose Conlon, "Half of Kansas nursing home investigator positions are vacant. Residents die waiting for help," *KCUR*, June 25, 2025, https://www.kcur.org/2025-06-25/kansas-nursing-home-investigator-positions-vacant-some-residents-die-waiting-for-help.

19 Ashley Borja, "Nearly Three in Four NYC Nursing Homes Haven't Been Inspected Within the Last 15 Months," *The City*, July 1, 2024, https://www.thecity.nyc/2024/07/01/nursing-home-inspections-abuses.

20 Miguel Faria-e-Castro and Samuel Jordan-Wood, "Excess Retirements Continue despite Ebbing COVID-19 Pandemic," *Federal Reserve Bank of St. Louis,* June 22, 2023, https://www.stlouisfed.org/on-the-economy/2023/jun/excess-retirements-covid19-pandemic#:~:text=As%20of%20April%202023%2C%20we%20estimate%20that%20there,rate%20since%20the%20recovery%20from%20the%20pandemic%20recession.

21 Jordan Reiland, "Why AHCA's Parkinson Predicts a Nursing Home Sector Recovery – And How to Get There," *Skilled Nursing News,* October 10, 2022, https://skillednursingnews.com/2022/10/why-ahcas-parkinson-predicts-a-nursing-home-sector-recovery-and-how-to-get-there.

Chapter III: The Truth Has Been Easy to Hide

22 "Couple booked 51 back-to-back cruises instead of retiring to a nursing home," *Cruise*, June 17, 2024, https://cruise.blog/2024/06/couple-booked-51-back-back-cruises-instead-retiring-nursing-home.

23 Foster Stubbs, "Could 'Golden Passport' tempt older adults to swap senior living for cruise ship living?," *McKnight's Senior Living*, August 27, 2025, https://www.mcknightsseniorliving.com/news/could-golden-passport-tempt-older-adults-to-swap-senior-living-for-cruise-ship-living/#:~:text=A%20new%20program%20from%20Villa%20Vie%20Residences%20offers,expert%2C%20but%20that's%20not%20necessarily%20cause%20for%20concern.

24 *Villa Vie Residences*, https://villavieresidences.com.

25 "Geriatrics and Extended Care," *U.S. Department of Veterans Affairs*, https://www.va.gov/geriatrics/pages/State_Veterans_Home_Program_Topics.asp.

26 "42 CFR Part 483 – Requirements for States and Long Term Care Facilities," *National Archives – Code of Federal Regulations*, https://www.ecfr.gov/current/title-42/chapter-IV/subchapter-G/part-483.

27 "Nursing Home Care Standards," *California Advocates for Nursing Home Reform*, October 24, 2022, https://canhr.org/nursing-home-care-standards.

28 "I'm getting Social Security benefits after 65," *Medicare.gov*, https://www.medicare.gov/basics/get-started-with-medicare/after-65.

29 "Understanding Medicare Advantage Plans," *Medicare.gov*, https://www.medicare.gov/publications/12026-understanding-medicare-advantage-plans.pdf.

30 Meredith Freed, Anthony Damico, Jeannie Fuglesten Biniek, and Tricia Neuman, "Medicare Advantage 2024 Spotlight: First Look," *KFF*, November 15, 2023, https://www.kff.org/medicare/medicare-advantage-2024-spotlight-first-look.

31 Meredith Freed, Jeannie Fuglesten Biniek, Anthony Damico, and Tricia Neuman, "Medicare Advantage in 2024: Enrollment Update and Key Trends," *KFF*, August 8, 2024, https://www.kff.org/medicare/medicare-advantage-in-2024-enrollment-update-and-key-trends.

32 "SilverSneakers for Seniors | Gyms Programs for Seniors," *Silver Sneakers*, https://tools.silversneakers.com/Eligibility/CheckEligibility?utm_source=bing&utm_medium=cpc&utm_term=gym%20programs%20for%20seniors&utm_campaign=sem_ss_b_nonbrand_pm_gyms&msclkid=2419c9f6a64d1ae98546a135a015f583.

33 "What Is the SilverSneakers Program," *Medicare.org*, June 4, 2025, https://www.medicare.org/articles/what-is-the-silversneakers-program.

34 "State of Medicare Advantage," *Better Medicare Alliance,* May 2021, https://bettermedicarealliance.org/wp-content/uploads/2021/05/BMA-State-of-MA-Report-2021.pdf.

35 "eHealth's Medicare Snapshot Report Highlights Plan Costs & Selection Trends from the First Half of Medicare's Annual Enrollment Period," *eHealth*, November 16, 2023, https://news.ehealthinsurance.com/news/ehealth-s-medicare-snapshot-report-highlights-plan-costs-selection-trends-from-the-first-half-of-medicare-s-annual-enrollment-period.

36 "Do Medicare Advantage Plans Follow CMS Guidelines?," *Medicare.org,* August 2, 2019, https://www.medicare.org/articles/do-medicare-advantage-plans-follow-cms-guidelines.

37 "Skilled Nursing Facility 3-Day Rule Billing," *CMS Medicare Learning Network,* May 2025, https://www.cms.gov/files/document/skilled-nursing-facility-3-day-rule-billing.pdf.

38 "Skilled nursing facility care," *Medicare.gov*, https://www.medicare.gov/coverage/skilled-nursing-facility-care.

39 Ibid.

40 "Leave Day Guidance," *Minnesota Department of Human Services*, April 10, 2016, https://mn.gov/dhs/assets/Leave-day-guidance_tcm1053-291451.pdf.

41 "Legislative Report Nursing Facility Rate Study Recommendation Report," *Minnesota Department of Human Services, Nursing Facility Rates and Policy Division*, May 2025, https://www.careproviders.org/Common/Uploaded%20files/Members/2025/Nursing_Facility_Rate_Study_DHS.pdf.

42 "15 Organizations Working to Advocate for Seniors," *SeniorAdvisor.com*, June 15, 2017, https://www.senioradvisor.com/blog/2017/06/15-organizations-working-to-advocate-for-seniors/?msockid=2ea21111437867d70b4003b542546601.

43 "Check Out These Organizations That Help Senior Citizens," *The Arbor Company*, https://www.arborcompany.com/blog/check-out-these-organizations-that-help-senior-citizens.

44 "Advocacy and Community," *AARP*, https://www.aarp.org/membership/benefits/community/#:~:text=Explore%20AARP%20member%20community%20resources.%20Get%20involved%20in,events%20and%20seminars%20to%20help%20boost%20your%20skills.?msockid=2ea21111437867d70b4003b542546601.

45 Kelly Maxwell, "17+ Important AARP Revenue and Membership Statistics In 2025," *Seniors Mutual*, December 14, 2024, https://seniorsmutual.com/aarp-statistics/#:~:text=AARP%20currently%20has%2038%20million%20members.%20The%20standard,over%202%20million%20members%20also%20die%20every%20year.

46 "About AARP," *AARP*, https://www.aarp.org/about-aarp/?msockid=2ea21111437867d70b4003b542546601.

47 "AARP Medicare Plans from United Healthcare," https://www.aarpmedicareplans.com.

48 "AARP Medicare Plans from United Healthcare," https://www.aarpmedicareplans.com/shop/medicare-supplement-plans.html.

49 "AARP Medicare Rx Plans from United Healthcare," AARP, https://www.aarp.org/membership/benefits/insurance/uhc-medicare-rx/?msockid=2ea21111437867d70b4003b542546601.

50 Chris Jacobs, "How AARP's Profits Harm Patients—And Violate Its Principles ," *Commitment to Seniors*, April 2024, https://commitmenttoseniors.org/wp-content/uploads/2024/04/April-2024-Chris-Jacobs-AARP-Report.pdf#:~:text=As%20it%20has%20grown%20and%20become%20more%20reliant,decades%20has%20come%20through%20its%20relationship%20with%20United-Health.

51 Ibid.

52 Ibid.

53 Ibid.

54 Meredith Freed, Jeannie Fuglesten Biniek, Anthony Damico, and Tricia Neuman, "Medicare Advantage in 2024: Enrollment Update and Key Trends," *KFF*, August 8, 2024, https://www.kff.org/medicare/medicare-advantage-in-2024-enrollment-update-and-key-trends.

Chapter IV: Life(style)-Sustaining Machinery

55 "Healthcare Programs," *U.S. Department of Housing and Urban Development*, https://www.hud.gov/hud-partners/healthcare-programs.

56 John O'Connor, "Hoping for God's grace is a dangerous business strategy," *McKnight's Long Term Care News,* August 30, 2025, https://www.mcknights.com/daily-editors-notes/hoping-for-gods-grace-is-a-dangerous-business-strategy.

57 Mariah Taylor, "California nursing home to pay $3.8M for physician referral scheme," *Becker's Hospital Review*, June 22, 2023, https://www.beckershospitalreview.com/post-acute/california-nursing-home-to-pay-3-8-for-physician-referral-scheme.

58 Ibid.

59 Kayla Jimenez, "California nursing facility agrees to pay $3.8 million for alleged kickbacks to doctors," *USA Today,* June 21, 2023, https://www.usatoday.com/story/news/nation/2023/06/21/alta-vista-healthcare-rockport-healthcare-services-pays-3-8-in-kickback-settlement/70344218007.

60 Ibid.

61 "Nursing Homes - ALTA VISTA HEALTHCARE & WELLNESS CENTRE, " *Healthcare Compare*, Updated March 12, 2019, https://healthcarecomps.com/nursing-homes/ca/055042.

62 *Alta Vista Healthcare and Wellness Centre*, 2025, https://www.altavistarehab.com.

63 "Tag Archives: Sacramento Bee," *BriusWatch.org*, https://briuswatch.org/tag/sacramento-bee.

64 "Facilities," *BriusWatch.org*, https://briuswatch.org/brius-facilities.

65 "South Florida Health Care Facility Owner Convicted for Role in Largest Health Care Fraud Scheme Ever Charged by The Department of Justice, Involving $1.3 Billion in Fraudulent Claims," *U.S. Department of Justice*, April 5, 2019, https://www.justice.gov/archives/opa/pr/south-florida-health-care-facility-owner-convicted-role-largest-health-care-fraud-scheme-ever#xd_co_f=ZTk2MzU4OWMtODgzOC00OGE1L-WE5ZjItNzQ2OTI0NzA1MTNm~.

66 Ibid.

67 Ibid.

68 Chris Pomorski, "Donald Trump Freed a Convicted Medicare Fraudster. The Justice Department Wants Him Back.," *Mother Jones*, November-December 2023, https://www.motherjones.com/politics/2023/11/philip-esformes-trial-morris-medicare-fraud-prosecution-donald-trump-clemency/.

69 Jay Weaver, "Miami healthcare exec Esformes sentenced to 20 years in biggest Medicare fraud case," Miami Herald, September 13, 2019, https://www.miamiherald.com/news/local/article234993252.html.

70 Chris Pomorski, "Donald Trump Freed a Convicted Medicare Fraudster. The Justice Department Wants Him Back.," *Mother Jones*, November-December 2023, https://www.motherjones.com/politics/2023/11/philip-esformes-trial-morris-medicare-fraud-prosecution-donald-trump-clemency/.

71 "United States of America vs. Philip Esformes, Government's Motion for Pre-Trial Detention and Supporting Memorandum," *U.S. District Court, Southern District* of Florida, July 22, 2016, https://www.justice.gov/archives/opa/file/878311/dl?inline=.

72 Paige Minemyer, "Florida health administrator charged in $1B fraud case," Fierce Healthcare, July 31, 2017, https://www.fiercehealthcare.com/finance/florida-health-administrator-charged-1b-fraud-case.

73 "United States of America vs. Philip Esformes, Government's Motion for Pre-Trial Detention and Supporting Memorandum," *U.S. District Court,*

Southern District of Florida, July 22, 2016, https://www.justice.gov/archives/opa/file/878311/dl?inline=.

74 Jay Weaver, "Wealthy Miami Beach executive charged anew with bribing state healthcare regulators," Miami Herald, February 13, 2017, https://www.miamiherald.com/news/local/article132038739.html.

75 Jay Weaver, "Miami healthcare exec Esformes sentenced to 20 years in biggest Medicare fraud case," Miami Herald, September 13, 2019, https://www.miamiherald.com/news/local/article234993252.html.

76 "United States of America vs. Philip Esformes, Government's Motion for Pre-Trial Detention and Supporting Memorandum," *U.S. District Court, Southern District* of Florida, July 22, 2016, https://www.justice.gov/archives/opa/file/878311/dl?inline=.

77 Jay Weaver, "Wealthy Miami Beach executive charged anew with bribing state healthcare regulators," Miami Herald, February 13, 2017, https://www.miamiherald.com/news/local/article132038739.html.

78 "United States of America v. Philip Esformes, Odette Barcha, and Arnaldo Carmouze - Indictment," *U.S. District Court, Southern District of Florida*, July 21, 2016, https://www.justice.gov/archives/opa/file/878306/dl.

79 Matthew Ormseth and Joel Rubin, "FBI found clues to college admissions scandal years earlier in massive Medicare fraud case," *Los Angeles Times*, July 26, 2019, https://www.latimes.com/california/story/2019-07-25/college-admissions-scandal-clues.

80 Jay Weaver, "Miami healthcare exec Esformes sentenced to 20 years in biggest Medicare fraud case," Miami Herald, September 13, 2019, https://www.miamiherald.com/news/local/article234993252.html.

81 Matthew Ormseth and Joel Rubin, "FBI found clues to college admissions scandal years earlier in massive Medicare fraud case," *Los Angeles Times*, July 26, 2019, https://www.latimes.com/california/story/2019-07-25/college-admissions-scandal-clues.

82 "United States of America v. Philip Esformes, Odette Barcha, and Arnaldo Carmouze - Indictment," *U.S. District Court, Southern District of Florida*, July 21, 2016, https://www.justice.gov/archives/opa/file/878306/dl.

Chapter V: Nursing Homes Struggle to Pass an Open Book Test

83 "State Operations Manual Appendix PP - Guidance to Surveyors for Long Term Care Facilities," *Centers for Medicare and Medicaid Services*, July 23, 2025 (Revised), https://www.cms.gov/regulations-and-guidance/guidance/manuals/downloads/som107ap_pp_guidelines_ltcf.pdf.

84 "Survey Summary," *Data.CMS.gov - Centers for Medicare and Medicaid Services*, July 30, 2025 (Released), https://data.cms.gov/provider-data/dataset/tbry-pc2d.

85 "Accreditation Pricing," *Joint Commission*, https://www.jointcommission.org/en-us/accreditation/pricing.

Chapter VI: Important People Don't Talk and Others Don't Listen

86 Lydia Saad, "Americans' Ratings of U.S. Professions Stay Historically Low," *Gallup*, January 13, 2025, https://news.gallup.com/poll/655106/americans-ratings-professions-stay-historically-low.aspx.

87 Jun Yan, "FDA Extends Black-Box Warning to All Antipsychotics," *Psychiatric News*, Volume 43, Number 14, July 18, 2008, https://psychiatryonline.org/doi/10.1176/pn.43.14.0001.

88 Dr Amrapali Bhandari, "A Study on the Impact of Performance Appraisal Systems on Employee Motivation and Career Progression," *International Journal of Education and Science Research Review*, Volume-6, Issue-2, March-April – 2019, https://ijesrr.org/publication/59/190.%20april%202019%20ijesrr.pdf., p.326.

89 "fulghum – All I Really Need To Know I Learned In Kindergarten (1989)," *Kerrisdale Gallery.com*, August 3, 2021, https://kerrisdalegallery.com/print/fulghum-all-i-really-need-to-know-i-learned-in-kindergarten-1989/fr089pv-fulghum-robert-all-i-really-need-to-know-i-learned-in-kindergarten-1989-poster-mgn.

Chapter VII: Agents of Change ... Aren't

90 Institute of Medicine (US) Committee on Nursing Home Regulation, "Improving the Quality of Care in Nursing Homes," *National Academies Press (US)*, 1986, https://www.ncbi.nlm.nih.gov/books/NBK217557.

91 "Distribution of Certified Nursing Facility Residents by Primary Payer Source," *KFF*, (2024), https://www.kff.org/state-health-policy-data/state-indicator/distribution-of-certified-nursing-facilities-by-primary-payer-source/?currentTimeframe=0&sortModel=%7B"colId":"Location","sort":"asc"%7D.

92 Tom J. Manos, "Florida's Nursing Home Reform and its Anticipated Effect on Litigation," *Florida Bar Journal,* Vol.75, No 11, December 2001, https://www.floridabar.org/the-florida-bar-journal/floridas-nursing-home-reform-and-its-anticipated-effect-on-litigation., p.18.

93 Denisse O. Gastélum, "Elder Abuse and Dependent Adult Civil Protection Act – Litigation 101," *Plaintiff Magazine*,

April 2020, https://plaintiffmagazine.com/recent-issues/item/elder-abuse-and-dependent-adult-civil-protection-act-litigation-101.

94 "Extendicare Health Services Inc. Agrees to Pay $38 Million to Settle False Claims Act Allegations Relating to the Provision of Substandard Nursing Care and Medically Unnecessary Rehabilitation Therapy," *Archives – U.S. Department of Justice,* October 10, 2014, https://www.justice.gov/archives/opa/pr/extendicare-health-services-inc-agrees-pay-38-million-settle-false-claims-act-allegations.

95 Tim Mullaney, "Extendicare to sell US businesses for $870 million," *McKnight's Long Term Care News*, November 10, 2014, https://www.mcknights.com/news/extendicare-to-sell-us-businesses-for-870-million.

96 Tim Mullaney, "Extendicare Closes $870 Million Sale of its U.S. Business to Formation," *Senior Housing News*, July 2, 2015, https://seniorhousingnews.com/2015/07/02/extendicare-closes-870-million-sale-of-its-u-s-business-to-formation/#:~:text=Canada-based%20Extendicare%20Inc.%20has%20completed%20the%20%24870%20million,LLC%2C%20effective%20July%201%2C%20the%20company%20announced%20today.

Chapter VIII: Big Thinkers, Small Ideas

97 "Bull Durham (1988) - Bunch of Lollygaggers Scene," *YouTube*, March 23, 2015, https://www.bing.com/videos/riverview/relatedvideo?q=bull+durham+lollygag+scene&&mid=2C6C6DCBCF296E5E14B52C6C6DCBCF296E5E14B5&FORM=VAMGZC.

98 Toby Edelman, "Special Report | Nursing Facilities Have Received Billions of Dollars in Direct Financial and Non-Financial Support During Coronavirus Pandemic," *Center for Medicare Advocacy*, March 17, 2021, https://medicareadvocacy.org/report-snf-financial-support-during-covid/.

99 Toby Edelman, "Paycheck Protection Program: A Massive Windfall for Nursing Facilities?," *Center for Medicare Advocacy*, August 3, 2023, https://medicareadvocacy.org/paycheck-protection-program-a-massive-windfall-for-nursing-facilities/.

100 "States' Backlogs of Standard Surveys of Nursing Homes Grew Substantially During the COVID-19 Pandemic," *U.S. Department of Health and Human Services, Office of Inspector General*, July 27, 2021, https://oig.hhs.gov/reports/all/2021/states-backlogs-of-standard-surveys-of-nursing-homes-grew-substantially-during-the-covid-19-pandemic/.

101 "Nursing Home Closures: By the Numbers," *American Health Care Association*, April 2022, https://www.ahcancal.org/News-and-Communications/Fact-Sheets/FactSheets/SNF-Closures-Report.pdf.

102 Priya Chidambaram and Alice Burns, "A Look at Nursing Facility Characteristics Between 2015 and 2024," *KFF*, December 4, 2024, https://www.kff.org/medicaid/a-look-at-nursing-facility-characteristics/.

103 Tim Mullaney, "'Tepid' Occupancy Recovery Continues with Flat Month for Post-Acute Care," *Skilled Nursing News*, April 23, 2023, https://skillednursingnews.com/2023/04/tepid-occupancy-recovery-continues-with-flat-month-for-post-acute-care/.

104 Danielle Brown, "Following record 2Q earnings, Ensign Group returns $110M in CARES Act funding," *McKnight's Long Term Care News,* August 7, 2020, https://www.mcknights.com/news/ensign-group-returns-110m-in-federal-relief-funding/.

105 Danielle Brown, "Ensign touts another record quarter, returns $23M in federal relief funding," *McKnight's Long Term Care News*, October 30, 2020, https://www.mcknights.com/news/ensign-touts-another-record-quarter-returns-23m-in-federal-relief-funding/.

106 Amy Stulick, ""Why Skilled Nursing Deal Volume Could be 'Exorbitant, Voluminous' in Back Half of 2023," *Skilled Nursing News*, June 27, 2023, https://skillednursingnews.com/2023/06/why-skilled-nursing-deal-volume-could-be-exorbitant-voluminous-in-back-half-of-2023/.

107 Robyn Stone, "Immigration Policies Must be Ethical and Equitable," *Leading Age LTSS Center @ UMass Boston,* September 25, 2023, https://www.ltsscenter.org/immigration-policies-must-be-ethical-and-equitable/.

108 "State of the world's nursing 2020: investing in education, jobs and leadership," *World Health Organ*ization, April 6, 2020, https://www.who.int/publications/i/item/9789240003279.

109 Ibid.

Chapter IX: Disruption Is Inevitable

110 Zoe Caplan, "U.S. Older Population Grew From 2010 to 2020 at Fastest Rate Since 1880 to 1890," *United States Census Bureau*, May 25, 2023, https://www.census.gov/library/stories/2023/05/2020-census-united-states-older-population-grew.html.

111 Jonathan Vespa, Lauren Medina, and David M. Armstrong, "Demographic Turning Points for the United States: Population Projections for 2020 to 2060," *United States Census Bureau*, Issued March 2018, Revised February 2020, https://www.census.gov/content/dam/Census/library/publications/2020/demo/p25-1144.pdf.

112 "2020 Profile of Older Americans", *The Administration for Community Living*, May 2021, https://acl.gov/sites/default/files/Aging%20and%20

Disability%20in%20America/2020ProfileOlderAmericans.Final_.pdf., pp.6-7.

113 Jenny Yang, "U.S. number of residents in certified nursing facilities as of 2024, by state," *Statista*, December 11, 2024, https://www.statista.com/statistics/1168843/number-residents-certified-nursing-facilities-state/.

114 "CMS Acts to Improve the Safety and Quality of Care of the Nation's Nursing Homes," *CMS.gov Newsroom*, July 29, 2022, https://www.cms.gov/newsroom/press-releases/cms-acts-improve-safety-and-quality-care-nations-nursing-homes.

115 Cara Stepanczuk, Alexandra Carpenter, Caitlin Murray, and Andrea Wysocki, Mathematica, "Medicaid Long-Term Services and Supports Users and Expenditures by Service Category, 2022," *Centers for Medicare and Medicaid Services*, August 29, 2024, https://www.medicaid.gov/medicaid/long-term-services-supports/downloads/ltss-users-expenditures-category-brief-2022.pdf.

116 "NHE Fact Sheet," *CMS.gov*, June 24, 2025, https://www.cms.gov/data-research/statistics-trends-and-reports/national-health-expenditure-data/nhe-fact-sheet.

117 Lydia Saad, "Americans Sour on U.S. Healthcare Quality," *Gallup*, January 19, 2023, https://news.gallup.com/poll/468176/americans-sour-healthcare-quality.aspx.

118 "NHE Fact Sheet," *CMS.gov*, June 24, 2025, https://www.cms.gov/data-research/statistics-trends-and-reports/national-health-expenditure-data/nhe-fact-sheet.

119 "Role of Body Weight in Osteoarthritis," *Johns Hopkins Arthritis Center*, https://www.hopkinsarthritis.org/patient-corner/disease-management/role-of-body-weight-in-osteoarthritis/.

120 S. Michaela Rikard, PhD· Andrea E. Strahan, PhD, Kristine M. Schmit, MD, Gery P. Guy Jr., PhD, "Chronic Pain Among Adults—United States, 2019–2021," *CDC Morbidity and Mortality Weekly Report*, April 14, 2023, 72(15), 379–385, https://www.cdc.gov/mmwr/volumes/72/wr/mm7215a1.htm.

121 Ibid.

122 "Where cannabis is legal in the United States," *The Cannigma*, April 2025, https://cannigma.com/us-states-where-cannabis-is-legal/.

123 Kenneth D. Kochanek, M.A., Sherry L. Murphy, B.S., Jiaquan Xu, M.D., and Elizabeth Arias, Ph.D., "Data Brief No. 492 - Mortality in the United States, 2022," *CDC – National Center for Health Statistics*, March 2024, https://www.cdc.gov/nchs/data/databriefs/db492.pdf.

124 "2024 Alzheimer's Disease Facts and Figures Report: Executive Summary," *Alzheimer's Association*, https://www.alz.org/getmedia/2421d513-8165-464a-a443-8ded08ae5b54/facts-and-figures-2024-executive-summary.pdf#:~:text=The%202024%20Alzheimer%27s%20Disease%20Facts%20and%20Figures%20report,costs%20of%20care.%20More%20Americans%20have%20Alzheimer's%20disease.

125 "Public Law 111–375—National Alzheimer's Project Act,.

126 Richard J. Hodes, "NAPA at 10: A decade of Alzheimer's and related dementias research progress," *National Institute on Aging*, May 16, 2022, https://www.nia.nih.gov/research/blog/2022/05/napa-at-10.

127 Heidi Mason, Mary Beth Derubeis, Beth Hesseltine, "Early Palliative Care for Oncology Patients: How APRNs Can Take the Lead," *Journal of Advanced Practice Oncology*, July 12, 2021, Volume 12, Number 5, p.477-484, https://www.advanced-practitioner.com/issues/volume-12-number-5-july-2021/early-palliative-care-for-oncology-patients-how-aprns-can-take-the-lead/.

128 "Medical Aid-In-Dying FAQs," *Completed Life Initiative*, https://completedlife.org/faqs/.

129 Stefanie Green, "This is Assisted Dying – A Doctor's Story of Empowering Patients at the End of Life, " (Simon & Schuster, 2022), p.45.

130 J. Arky, "US States With the Most (and the Least) Debt," *GO Banking Rates*, November 29, 2023, https://www.gobankingrates.com/money/economy/states-with-the-most-least-debt/.

131 Kimberly Marselas, "State forces nursing home rate cut, raising doubts about ability to provide required services," *McKnight's Long Term Care News*, August 26, 2025, https://www.mcknights.com/news/state-forces-nursing-home-rate-cut-raising-doubts-about-ability-to-provide-required-services/.

132 Andrew Wilford, "Interstate Migration in Minutes: How Fast Are Taxpayers Leaving or Entering Each State?", *National Taxpayers Union Foundation*, November 24, 2025, https://www.ntu.org/foundation/detail/interstate-migration-in-minutes-how-fast-are-taxpayers-leaving-or-entering-each-state.

133 "Status of the Social Security and Medicare Programs - A Summary of the 2024 Annual Reports," *Social Security and Medicare Boards of Trustees*, https://www.ssa.gov/OACT/TRSUM/tr24summary.pdf.

134 Ibid.

135 Ibid.

136 "2. Americans' views of government aid to poor, role in health care and Social Security," *Pew Research Center*, June 24, 2024, https://www.pewre-

search.org/politics/2024/06/24/americans-views-of-government-aid-to-poor-role-in-health-care-and-social-security/.

137 "Rural Hospitals At Risk of Closing," *Center for Healthcare Quality and Payment Reform*, August 2025, https://chqpr.org/downloads/Rural_Hospitals_at_Risk_of_Closing.pdf.

138 "Healthcare Restructuring: Trends and Outlook Analysis of Chapter 11 Healthcare Bankruptcies since 2019 Interim 2025 Report," *Gibbins Advisors*, August 5, 2025, https://static1.squarespace.com/static/6806e9b-b1a73e928f078432d/t/689e6c04ec85721dc700443c/1755212804495/Gibbins+Advisors+Healthcare+Bankruptcies+Interim+2025+Report-Final.pdf.

139 "Mental Health By the Numbers," *National Alliance on Mental Illness*, https://www.nami.org/about-mental-illness/mental-health-by-the-numbers/.

140 "Highlights from the 2022 National Survey on Drug Use and Health," *Substance Abuse and Mental Health Services Administration*, 2023, https://www.samhsa.gov/data/sites/default/files/reports/rpt42731/2022-nsduh-main-highlights.pdf.

141 Kilmer G, Omura JD, Bouldin ED, et al., "Changes in Health Indicators Among Caregivers—United States, 2015–2016 to 2021–2022," *Morbidity and Mortality Weekly Report*, August 29, 2024;73:740–746. DOI: http://dx.doi.org/10.15585/mmwr.mm7334a2.

Chapter X; Disruption Is Here

142 "Lennar Loves Home, " Le*nnar Homes*, July 7, 2025, https://resourcecenter.lennar.com/our-communities/discover-next-gen-a-new-way-of-living/.

143 "Lennar Full Year 2024 Earnings: In Line With Expectations, *Simply Wall Street*, January 25, 2025, https://finance.yahoo.com/news/lennar-full-2024-earnings-line-142631578.html.

144 "Home is Where the Hospital Is, " *Johns Hopkins Bloomberg School of Public Health,* December 7. 2005, https://publichealth.jhu.edu/2005/burton-hospital-home.

145 Amy Berman, "Hartford Foundation and CMMI Work Together to Spread Hospital at Home Model," *The John A. Hartford Foundation*, November 13, 2014, https://www.johnahartford.org/blog/view/hartford-foundation-and-cmmi-work-together-to-spread-hospital-at-home-model/.

146 "Understanding the Hospital At Home Program," *American Hospital Association*, https://www.aha.org/system/files/media/file/2024/08/understanding-the-hospital-at-home-program-infographic.pdf.

147 "Report on the Study of the Acute Hospital Care at Home Initiative,"

Centers for Medicare and Medicaid Services, September, 2024, https://qualitynet.cms.gov/files/66fae9162702fb414b540545?filename=AHCAH_Study_092724.pdf.

148 Andrew Donlan, "CMS Hospital-at-Home Program Closing In On 200 Participants," *Home Health Care News*, April 19, 2021, https://homehealthcarenews.com/2021/04/cms-hospital-at-home-program-closing-in-on-200-participants/.

149 "Report on the Study of the Acute Hospital Care at Home Initiative," *Centers for Medicare and Medicaid Services*, September, 2024, https://qualitynet.cms.gov/files/66fae9162702fb414b540545?filename=AHCAH_Study_092724.pdf.

150 "Fact Sheet: Extending the Hospital-at-Home Program," *American Hospital Association*, July 2025, https://www.aha.org/fact-sheets/2024-08-06-fact-sheet-extending-hospital-home-program.

151 "Amedisys Acquires Contessa Health for $250 Million," *Bass, Berry + Sims*, https://www.bassberry.com/experience/amedisys-acquires-contessa-health-for-250-million/.

152 Jim Parker, "Optum Fuels Growth for UnitedHealth Group with Amedisys Deal in the Wings," *Hospice Care News*, July 17, 2024, https://hospicenews.com/2024/07/17/optum-fuels-growth-for-unitedhealth-group-with-amedisys-deal-in-the-wings/.

153 Ibid.

154 Haleluya Hadero, "Amazon gets FAA approval allowing it to expand drone deliveries for online orders," *AP News*, May 30, 2024, https://apnews.com/article/amazon-drone-delivery-faa-texas-41e663b3fcc25f5190b982c0963f646d.

155 Clifford Stoll, "The Internet, Bah!" *Newsweek*, February 26, 1995, Updated: April 19, 2023, https://www.newsweek.com/clifford-stoll-why-web-wont-be-nirvana-185306.

156 Ibid.

ABOUT THE AUTHOR

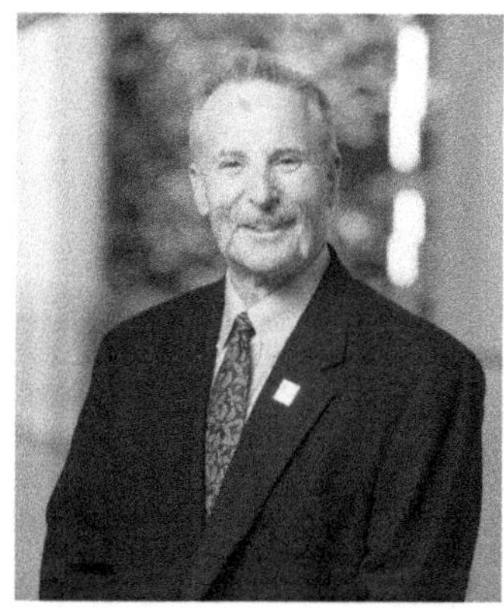

Dave Devereaux is a nationally recognized leader in the field of long-term care, with a career spanning more than 45 years of service, innovation, and advocacy. From his early days as a teenage housekeeper in a nursing home to senior executive roles overseeing multi-state healthcare organizations, Dave has dedicated his career to improving systems of care and the lives of those they serve.

He holds a B.S. from Cornell University and an M.B.A. from Temple University. Beyond his professional accomplishments, Dave is known for his philanthropic vision and enduring commitment to education and healthcare delivery. He endowed the Chair of Temple University's Nursing Department in 2006, established the Visionary Research Fund for Temple's College of Public Health in 2012, and, together with his wife, founded the University of Georgia Music Therapy Graduate Fellowship.

In recognition of his leadership and impact, Dave was named a Centennial Honoree by Temple University's Fox School of Business in 2018.

A native of northeastern Pennsylvania, Dave now resides in the South with his wife, Patrice, continuing to inspire innovation and compassion across the long-term care community.

For more information go to: www.davedevereaux.com